1991

Indices of Quality
in Long-Term Care:
Research and Practice

Pub. No. 20-2292

National League for Nursing

Contents

Foreword

Our society is being challenged to find cost-effective ways to provide quality long-term care for our chronically ill, aging population. Even as the older adult population increases, we recognize that resources to care for this population are limited. The government and third party payers are increasingly discerning about what they will and will not pay for. Reimbursement policies have been based on a medical model focusing on short-term care. A new model that focuses on long-term care and on health rather than on illness is needed. Additionally, the existing nursing shortage presents a serious challenge in the face of increasing acuity of long-term care patients. How do we recruit adequate numbers of nurses to provide the quality of care needed?

Quality has become a key word. What kind of care is the highest quality and can result in the best patient outcomes? Who can provide this care most effectively? Which patients will benefit most from community-based home care and which will be most effectively cared for in a nursing home setting? How do we measure quality?

Increasingly, we are recognizing the need to define and measure quality in long-term care. Research in both the community home care setting and the nursing home setting is essential to identify meaningful, valid patient outcomes. This conference, "Indices of Quality in Long-Term Care," represents a timely and comprehensive overview of some of the research already done in this area, research that is still in process, and most importantly, those questions that still need to be answered. We hope that publication of the following papers will trigger ideas and action for future research. It is essential for nursing and other health care professionals to present valid research data to develop a new model of health care. This model would identify quality health care in the long-term care arena and would be a realistic basis for reimbursement systems.

v

It has been an honor and a pleasure to work with the National League for Nursing Long-Term Care Committee in facilitating this invitational conference.

Sherry Bockus, MS, RN
Director, Medical Nutritional Nursing Services,
Ross Laboratories

Jim McCall, FACHCA
Director, Organizational Services,
Ross Laboratories

Introduction

We began the first series of invitational conferences with a vision of constructing models for nursing education, service, and research that would help to overcome the bias of ageism in our society and our profession. The focus was on long-term care of the elderly in a variety of settings, with an emphasis on the fact that close to 95 percent of the 65 plus population either care for themselves or live with relatives, and they strive to gain access to support services that will avoid institutionalization. Somewhere, we felt, between the ideal and the real are the essentials for quality living in the institutional and in the home setting. Familial care and concern would require the support of a continuum of services that could change and adjust to meet the needs of patients and families as they shifted.

Our discussions clearly recognized the need for innovation and the cost involved in improving the care delivery system. Inherent in all of the deliberations was an overriding concern for quality care and quality living.

As we move into the second five-year series of invitational conferences, the agenda will focus on the indices of quality in service, education, research, and public policy. In this connection, future conferences will involve the recipients of long-term care in the dialogue so we can begin to understand their viewpoint and factor the patient's perspective into any discussion of quality or endeavors to identify quality outcomes of care. For too long our discussions around quality issues have been fraught with contradictions; and we are trapped into believing that our practices and interventions are for the patients own good. Yet the patient is conspicuously left out of the dialogue. We need to examine alternative care practices that truly take the patient perspective into account. The achievement of quality from the patient view may require us to change our mindset.

Quality, defined by the recipients of care, will indeed require accrediting bodies and government surveyors alike to change their approach to quality and focus on a wider variety of interpretations as to what quality of life and care are all about. This is our challenge for the future.

The conference held in Scottsdale, Arizona, January 1989, discussed the relationship between research in long-term care and the quality of service.

Participants in the discussions experienced the all too common frustration of being unable to identify research findings that have been transformed into practice. Thanks to Barbara K. Haight, DrPh, RNC and Sr. Rose Therese Bahr, PhD, RN, FAAN, a Delphi Study, funded by the College of Nursing, Gerontological Nursing Graduate Program, Medical University of South Carolina, has been developed to identify a research agenda for Long-Term Care in the 1990s.

We have high expectations for an outcome-oriented process that will aid us in achieving a high degree of quality of life for those of us who do receive or will receive long-term care as part of our life experience.

Sr. Anne Marie McNicholl, PhD, RN, RPT
Chairperson
Ross Laboratories/National League for Nursing Long-Term Care
Invitational Conference

1

Long-Term Care

Maria K. Mitchell, MS, RN, CPNP
Senior Vice President
Community Health Accreditation Program
National League for Nursing
New York, NY

There is no more pressing problem in our health care system today than what to do about long-term care. A glance at almost any magazine or newspaper in this country can reveal the extent and depth of the problem facing us. Although we have known the state of disarray in which long-term care has existed for some time, precious little has been done to ameliorate this disarray or address the problems directly.

Several years ago, I had a unique opportunity to see the full extent and depth of the problem. This opportunity did not stem from the direct source, care of long-term patients, but from a broader policy perspective.

While working in New York City government and heading the Mayor's Interagency Task Force on AIDS, which was responsible for coordinating the efforts of each of the city's four health-related agencies in serving persons with AIDS (Health and Hospitals Corporation (HHC), Human Resources Administration (HRA), Department of Health (DOH), and Department of Mental Health (DMH)) it became immediately clear that AIDS actually served to crystalize the myriad problems in the health care system itself. In fact, it became apparent that there really was no system in place at all. More specifically, and for our purposes here, there was no national system of long-term care.

1

People became infected with AIDS and, most often, suffered the onset of acute illnesses simply because there was no primary care system to diagnose them early. As a result, they were hospitalized. Such hospital stays were long and costly. By the time these patients were ready for discharge from the hospital, they usually needed some form of after care. But out-of-hospital care was rarely available to them. To compound this problem, neither coverage for home care nor nursing home beds for AIDS patients existed (for the most part, they still don't). AIDS patients had the opportunity to wait two years for Medicare disability, but few of them (at that time) lived for the required two-year period. Even hospice care wasn't an option for these patients because they did not meet the appropriate reimbursement criteria; they had already spent too many days in the hospital. Again, this was compounded by the fact that hospital discharge planners had little knowledge of the availability of services for AIDS patients and almost no one understood the financing of the system. It soon became clear that this situation was not unique to AIDS patients; Alzheimer's patients had similar problems, as did thousands of other patients needing out-of-hospital care. In fact, there was really little difference in what people with AIDS were experiencing than most chronically ill people in our society. The problem of caring for AIDS patients was not so much the disease but the health care system itself. The fact that there were so many young, vital, and creative people dying merely jolted us into finally examining this system, or lack of one.

When we examine long-term care, beginning with discharge planning at hospitals to nursing homes, to home care, to hospice care, we do not see a continuum that serves the people it is intended to serve, but an extraordinarily fragmented and disorganized system, with numerous individuals falling between the cracks and many shuttled to the wrong level of care. This has occurred because long-term care is not a system based on *need* but *affordability*. For the most part, finances have shaped our long-term care system.

As a result, then, of reimbursement technicalities and a system so confusing that perhaps only its architects understand it, patients often are discharged to an inappropriate level of care, or they don't have the appropriate level of caregiver. Therefore, either long-term care patients don't reach the desired outcome or they do so in a longer period of time than necessary, and costs escalate. How we address these problems is symptomatic of a failure in the system itself. We look at costs to the exclusion of quality, the cycle continues, and the system does not improve.

On top of all this, we know that actual service delivery often leaves much to be desired. Aside from the fact that it is impossible to receive the proper care in such a fragmented system, the state of our long-term care facilities, by and large, do not achieve a passing grade. The results of the recent *Consumer*

Guide to Quality in Nursing Homes were somewhat frightening. According to this guide, our nursing homes are barely able to assure that their residents receive even basic services. Nearly 30 percent of the nation's nursing homes failed to meet the standard under the daily, personal hygiene category, which includes cleanliness, good skin care, good grooming, and oral hygiene. Forty-two percent of nursing homes failed to meet standards of food storage, refrigeration , sanitation, and preparation of food.

This means, according to the government, that in nearly half of the nursing homes in this country, we can't be certain that our family members will be properly fed and bathed. Such uncertainty regarding only basic health care measures, after months of fighting to get a family member into the system to begin with, is shocking. It is little wonder that the general public's image of nursing homes is so poor.

To date, the only real response to such an inequitable system has been more government regulation. Yet, in long-term care, government regulation has not even begun to approach the elementary level of trying to define and measure quality itself. In fact, federal regulation has not progressed beyond trying to assure minimum safety requirements. But, as the above statistics testify, even this attempt has failed. The government is still trying to make sure that people are fed and bathed properly.

In 1863 Florence Nightingale said that "The first requirement of a hospital is that it should do the sick no harm." In long-term care, we've just about fulfilled this first requirement. However, when do we begin to take a comprehensive look at real quality? In this regard, I don't believe you can expect much from the federal government.

With the federal deficit looming over the Bush administration and a vow not to raise taxes, there will be fewer and fewer resources devoted to health care quality concerns. In fact, in this week's *Newsweek*, an article on long-term care states, "Of all the medical spending issues facing Americans, long-term health care most deeply troubles the heart."

Even consumer organizations committed to advancing quality health care for the elderly are concerned that, while government regulations might actually increase, there isn't enough money to assure quality. In addition, real concern has been expressed that the federal government would not be able to properly fund a long-term care quality initiative. As a result, and as the Bush administration has been saying, it might be time for a public/private partnership to assure that the job gets done.

The question remains, what are we in the long-term care industry going to do to solve this problem? In particular, what is the nursing profession going to do? Unfortunately, if we do nothing, we can be certain that the federal government *will* do something. No doubt more ineffective regulations will be set forth. Furthermore, if nursing does nothing, the federal government will align itself with another professional group, and it is more than likely that this group will be physicians.

And as it occurred in the hospital industry where nurses were conspicuously left out of the standards setting process, nurses, again, will not be involved in setting standards for care and nursing practice in the long-term care arena. A long-term care industry will result where the experts of care will not have set the standards. Those professionals most intimately involved with patients—nurses—will be kept farthest away from determining what quality care is all about. If this occurs, we can be certain that true quality will never be attained in long-term care.

If nurses have nothing to say about setting standards in a system that delivers predominantly nursing care, then, regardless of how high a standard one aspires to, its implementation will be fraught with impotence. We need only to look at the hospital industry to know that this is the case. Nurses did not set the standards for practice in the hospital and there is constant discontent in the nursing community regarding their role in the hospital, to say nothing of the severe nursing shortage we now face.

Finally, however, nurses have an unprecedented opportunity to seize the initiative and truly reshape the long-term care system into a system relevant and responsive to patients' needs. Nurses must also ensure that the long-term care system is driven by *quality*, and not *financial*, concerns.

An industry that consists of predominantly nursing practice should be governed by nurses. Standards of care should be set by nurses. Together with the federal government and consumers of care, nurses should forge a public/private partnership for long-term care using an approach similar to what we at the National League for Nursing are using in home care with our subsidiary, the Community Health Accreditation Program (CHAP).

In CHAP, we have taken a major departure from the status quo to assure quality through accreditation in the home care industry. Let me explain:

The National League for Nursing has been accrediting home care organizations since 1965. In 1987, CHAP became a fully independent subsidiary of NLN. CHAP was created as a subsidiary primarily because of NLN's commitment to quality and the belief that quality can only be achieved by meeting the needs of the consumer. Therefore, the Board of Directors of CHAP are consumers, including business and insurance representatives as well as individual consumers and providers.

CHAP's philosophy is founded on the basic principle that a voluntary commitment to excellence by home care and community health organizations is the only way to assure the availability of quality community based health care services. CHAP's purpose is to establish consumer-oriented, state-of-the-art standards or excellence which are applied through a mechanism to assist participating organizations, and which will elevate the quality and strengthen the long-term viability of community based health care overall. The CHAP accreditation process is unique in that the approach is consultative rather than punitive. CHAP site visitors point out strengths as well as weaknesses while providing clear direction for improvement. In an effort to assure that consumers have access to information necessary to make informed decisions regarding home care, CHAP also has a detailed policy on public disclosure.

Instead of a fragmented and disorganized system driven by reimbursement, a system that fails to serve the very people it aims to serve, we should continue with the development of quality indicators, not just in home care, but in long-term care as well, from a managed care perspective. As the primary caregivers in long-term care, we should assure that reliabile quality indicators drive a managed long-term care system that meets the needs of all its intended recipients, along the entire continuum of care, from hospitals to nursing homes, to home care.

Because the system is in such disarray, and because of the servere nursing shortage, national attention is focused on the nursing profession. Consumers are looking to nursing to help solve these problems. We must seize the initiative before it slips from our grasp. The worst of times can become the best of times for nursing. The system's greatest problem—quality in long-term care—remains nursing's greatest strength.

2

Update on Research in Long-Term Care: 1984–1988

Barbara K. Haight, DrPH, RNC
Associate Professor
College of Nursing
Medical University of South Carolina
Charleston, SC

NURSING RESEARCH IN LONG-TERM CARE FACILITIES
(1984–1988)

This paper focuses on nursing research in long-term care facilities from 1984–1988. Specifically, four areas are discussed: past reviews of gerontological nursing research, findings from a current search of nursing research in long-term care facilities, current trends, and suggestions for future research. Additionally, an integrated review of five years of research in long-term care facilities is presented in Appendix I.

Past Reviews of Research

Irene Burnside (1985) reviewed the gerontological nursing research literature for a National League for Nursing Long-Term Care Conference. In her review, Burnside synthesized four previous overviews and research critiques (Basson,

7

1967; Gunter & Miller, 1977; Robinson, 1981; Kayser-Jones, 1981). These early critiques identified serious deficiencies in the research at that time, including an absence of theoretical frameworks and the use of rigid research designs.

Another shortcoming was the propensity of nurse researchers to study attitudes among nurses and student nurses to the exclusion of other topics. Additionally, an emphasis on the psychosocial needs of patients, rather than the physical needs of patients, further characterized gerontological nursing research until the 1980s. Table 1 reflects these limitations of gerontological nursing research identified in the first four reviews.

Table 1
Limitations of Gerontological Research

No theoretical frameworks.
Problem solving research only.
No health promotion and disease prevention studies.
Few studies based on physical science.
No longitudinal studies.

In her later review covering 1979–1984, Burnside noted improvements in nurses' research and determined that nurses increasingly used theoretical frameworks as the basis for their research. She also discovered other improvements, including use of tighter designs and collaboration with other disciplines. However, nurses' seemingly main interest in attitudes and psychosocial nursing research continued, and nursing research into the physical areas of care continued to be neglected. At the same time, there remained a scarcity of scholarly inquiry about the elderly by nursing writers other than gerontological nurse researchers.

From her review, Burnside presented 28 subject areas still requiring the attention of nurse researchers. Burnside also documented a report by Benedict (1975) suggesting the need to conduct evaluation studies of specific nursing home care topics, including:

1. Discharge and admission of residents (source of patients, frequency and appropriateness of admission, and post-discharge care).

2. Responsibilities of nurses and physicians (incident reports, use of nurses for non-nursing functions, physician visits, and common diagnoses).

3. Nursing care (weight loss, bowel and bladder training, care of the dying).

4. Drugs (medication and diet, adequacy of policies and procedures for medication, and drug interactions).

Most topics identified by Burnside and Benedict still have not been researched, and opportunities remain for nurse researchers in gerontology. The need for research, particularly in long-term care, is overwhelming. Table 2 presents these subject areas.

Table 2
Burnside's Areas of Concern

Abuse	Intensive care unit syndrome
Alzheimer's disease and care	Life review therapy
Catastrophic reactions	Living arrangements
Confidants	Nutrition
Cost-effective deliveries or therapies	Paranoia
Delirium and dementia	Pet therapy
Depression	Reminiscence therapy
Exercise and mobility	Restraints
Health centers for elderly, nurse managed	Self-esteem
Hearing problems	Sensory deprivation or overload
Hypothermia and hyperthermia	Significant others
Incontinence	Suicide
Infection control	Sundowner's syndrome
	Visual problems
	Wandering behavior

From National League for Nursing. (1986). *Overcoming the bias of ageism in long-term care.* New York: National League for Nursing, p. 134.

Current Research Review (1984–1988)

Journals Searched. The current literature search examined five years of gerontological nursing research in long-term care facilities. The three major research journals and two gerontology journals selected for this review were: the *Journal of Gerontological Nursing, Geriatric Nursing, Nursing Research, Research in Nursing and Health,* and the *Western Journal of Nursing Research.* The *Journal of Gerontological Nursing* published most of the research (47 articles). Unfortunately, research articles in this journal generally lacked a theoretical basis and a stringent research format and did not provide enough information to replicate the studies. However, the pieces were well written and generally interesting, providing many ideas for practice in nursing homes.

Geriatric Nursing, a clinical journal, contributed only 10 studies. Most studies in this journal were clinically derived and, therefore, useful in the clinical setting. The study that was least clinically based discussed relocation (Amenta, Weiner, & Amenta, 1984). A few select examples of clinically based studies follow: Pearson and Droessler (1988) studied incontinence. Adams (1988) and Gaspar (1988) addressed fluid intake while Blom (1985) reported on a three-year quality assurance program that reduced the incidence of decubiti by 81 percent.

The three major research journals, *Nursing Research, Research in Nursing and Health*, and the *Western Journal of Nursing Research*, provided a total of seven reports on nursing research in nursing homes. These articles employed a strict research format and were based on theory. The results were applicable to clinical practice in nursing homes. Selected topics included functional assessment (Travis, 1988), cognitive assessment (Roberts & Lincoln, 1988), treatment of decubiti (Diekmann, 1984), and situational control (Ryden, 1984 & 1985).

Of these three journals, *Research in Nursing and Health* published the greatest number of research studies in long-term care. In contrast, the *Western Journal of Nursing Research* did not contribute to the literature on research in nursing homes during the entire five-year period. Table 3 presents the journals searched and their contributions.

Table 3
Research in Long-Term Care by Publication 1984–1988

Journal	Number of Articles
Journal of Gerontological Nursing	47
Geriatric Nursing	10
Journal of Nursing Research	3
Research and Health in Nursing	4
Western Journal of Nursing Research	0
Total	64

Topic Areas and Trends. An analysis of the articles in the five-year literature search served to separate them into topic areas. New trends emerged when placing these articles into categories. For example, nurse researchers finally discarded their emphasis on attitudes of nurses and nursing students toward the elderly. The 1984–1988 search disclosed only three studies focusing on attitudes in nursing home settings (Gomez, Otto, Blattstein, & Gomez, 1985; Winger & Smyth-Staruch, 1986; Heller, Bausell, & Ninos, 1984). Nurses appeared to be shifting toward researching physical problems. Studies of incontinence, pressure sores, and food and fluid intake illustrate this new and important trend.

Eight studies dealt with incontinence (Whitman & Kursh, 1987; Haeker, 1985; Long, 1985; Pearson & Droessler, 1988; Burgio, Jones, & Engle, 1988; Ouslander, Morishita, Blaustein, Orzeck, Dunn, & Sayre, 1987). Two of the incontinence studies by Yu (1987) (one with Kaltreider, 1987) investigated stress in both staff and patients when dealing with incontinence. Whitman et al. (1987) looked at the result of nursing and medical interventions on eight incontinent patients in a nursing home. The medical intervention diagnosed urinary tract infections in 50 percent of the patients while five of the eight patients presented with neurogenic bladder. The research showed that treatment of incontinence resulted in a 75 percent improvement rate, clearly indicating the capability and need to treat this condition.

Four studies examined food and fluid intake (Gaspar 1988; Michaelsson, Norberg, & Norberg, 1987; Adams 1988; Eaton, Mitchell-Bonair, & Friedmann, 1986). Touch as separate independent variable (Eaton et al., 1986) had a significant positive effect on the nutritional intake of organic brain syndrome patients. As a symbol of caring, touch should influence care givers to consider mealtime a caring, social event rather than a time to accomplish a task. Both staff and patients will benefit from an improved meal atmosphere.

Five more studies addressed pressure sores (Blom, 1985; Pajk, Craven, Cameron, Shipps, & Bennun, 1986; Bristow, Goldfarb, & Green, 1987; Boykin & Winland-Brown, 1986; Diekmann, 1984), with three of these studies based on interventions. Only one intervention, however, the use of the Clinitron bed, was successful. Two other interventions, saline irrigation and hydrocolloid occlusive dressings, proved ineffective. However, the use of this knowledge will save time, effort, and money in nursing homes by mitigating the use of ineffective interventions.

Other necessary areas of inquiry are nursing intervention studies. Practicing nurses value studies focusing on interventions because they have practical uses. Six of the studies scrutinized nursing interventions conducted in the long-term care setting. Two studies explored the innovative use of plush animals. Milton and MacPhail (1985) concluded that the use of stuffed animals should not be labeled as infantilism. In addition, Francis and Baly (1986) established that stuffed animals increased self-esteem, psychological well being, and life satisfaction.

Another nursing intervention study reported slow stroke back rub as contributing to relaxation (Fakouri & Jones, 1987). Again, touch proved valuable as an intervention increasing oral response in the elderly (Hollinger, 1986). Last, Lappe (1987) tested the intervention of reminiscing in groups. She determined that a 10-week reminiscing group offered once-a-week increased well being equal to a group offered twice a week.

While physically based research increased, research on psychosocial well being was not ignored. The psychosocial literature looked at aspects of communication and interaction between patients and staff. Along with communication, researchers studied the behavior of patients. For example, Roberts and Lincoln (1988) looked at variables that caused cognitive disturbance in hospitals and institutions, while Burgio, Jones, Butler, and Engle (1988) actually observed the occurrence of behavior problems in institutions.

Unfortunately, other needed areas of inquiry were overlooked, such as the continuing scrutiny of Alzheimer's disease. In five years of research, journals published only two nursing studies of Alzheimer's patients. One study by Hussian and Brown (1987) effectively used visual grid patterns to present a barrier to wandering Alzheimer's patients. Though the sample size was small, the study is valuable and needs replication. In another study useful for nursing care, Doyle, Dunn, Thadani, and Lenihan (1986) surveyed the functional ability of Alzheimer's victims.

The largest category of nursing research was listed as *other*. Eleven studies were too individually different to categorize and dealt with problems such as thermal regulation (Wirtz, 1987), learned helplessness (Slimmer, Lopez, LeSage, & Ellor, 1987), dress and self-esteem (Pensiero & Adams, 1987), documentation (Petrucci, McCormick, & Scheve, 1987), patient acuity level (Stull & Vernon, 1986), time experience (Strumpf, 1986), decision making (Sloane, Lekan-Rutledge, & Gilchrist, 1986), examination of small bore feeding tubes as cause of infection (Pritchard, 1988), situational control (Ryden, 1984 & 1985), and taste (Spitzer, 1988). Thirteen additional categories are arranged according to topic in the integrated review in the appendix. Table 4 illustrates the relationship of topics to number of articles published.

Table 4
Research in Nursing Homes by Topic 1984–1988

Topic	Number of Articles
Other	11
Incontinence	8
Nursing intervention	6
Assessment functional	6
Food and fluids	5
Pressure sores	5
Behavior	4
Communication and interaction	3
Falls	3
Relocation	4
Attitude	3
Confusion.	2
Drugs	2
Sleep	2
Alzheimer's	2

Suggestions for the Future

Analysis of the foregoing indicates that additional aspects of nursing home care require research. Thus, suggestions for future research have been categorized and these suggestions along with the needs identified by Burnside (1985) provide a complete research agenda for the 1990's. Three of these potential topics—research utilization, end-stage Alzheimer's disease, and nursing home environment—will be discussed in some detail as examples for the entire list. Table 5 outlines a recommended draft of potential topics.

Table 5
Future Research Needs

Environment	Health Promotion and Clinical Problems	Disease Prevention
Wheel chairs	Apathy	Exercise
Bathing facilities	Depression	Recreational activities
Single rooms	Treatments	(meaningful)
Safety features	Restraints	Counseling
Wandering paths	Hip fracture	Infection control
Outside extenders	Immobility	Functional ability
Roommates	Alzheimer's	Goal setting
Recliners—other chairs	End-stage of Alzheimer's	Work responsibilities
Bathing facilities	CVAer	
Lighting	COPD	
Quiet rooms	Grieving	
	Vascular problems	

Staff and Costs	Patient and Family	Nursing Practice
Staff patterns and models	Function	Protocols
Use of clinical nurse specialist	Grief	Nursing diagnosis
Use of aide	Orientation	Regulations versus care
Education of staff	Counseling	Computer use
Primary nursing	Treatment team	Quality assurance
Team nursing	Classification schemes	
Screening attitudes	Respite care	
Delivery of care		
Varied levels of care		

Research Utilization. Effective use and evaluation of completed research comprise the next development in upgrading nursing home care. Of the 65 studies reviewed, at least 50 provided useful information for nurses in practice.

Each reported study was reviewed in a subjective manner for immediate and useful application in the nursing home setting.

However, today's nursing home staffing patterns do not provide for the implementation of nursing research. With one nurse to a nursing home each 24-hour period, there is little thought to the use of research in actual practice. Perhaps utilization of research is a role for the clinical nurse specialist. To actually use research in nursing homes, one person must remain current with the research literature and then translate the research studies into useful pieces for nursing home application. The halo effect of current research programs alone will improve nursing care in model homes that use nursing research. Costing-out benefits of research projects may convince nursing home owners and administrators to practice nursing research in their facilities as well.

Obviously, these results need to be shared. One way to do this is to distribute a free newsletter, stating the concise results and directions for application in other nursing home settings.

Alzheimer's Disease.   The effective nursing care of the Alzheimer's victim is the next suggested area of inquiry. Barry Reisberg (1983) fully described the first seven stages of Alzheimer's disease. This staging helped caregivers determine the needs of the Alzheimer's victim as the disease progressed. However, Reisberg's research, and other's, ends at the beginning of the last stage. The last stage often finds the victims in nursing homes where, obviously, the quality of custodial care varies. Nursing must examine this last stage of the disease to ascertain the best technique for the most favorable care.

One research suggestion for nursing is to closely examine the care needed in the end stage of Alzheimer's disease to provide the highest quality of life. For example, Reisberg (1983) likens his seven stages of Alzheimer's disease to the reverse stages of childhood, moving from adolescence back to infanthood. If the final stage of Alzheimer's is similar to infancy, can nursing learn new approaches to the care of this Alzheimer's victim by searching the literature on infant care? For example, if the end-stage Alzheimer's victim is restless, the victim may need to be wrapped in blankets, just as an infant is swaddled, to gain comfort, warmth, and security. To take this approach, nurses must put aside beliefs that such care speaks of infantilism and be open to alternative modes of care. Through research, the nurse can continually find new ways to improve the quality of life of the Alzheimer's victim.

Nursing Home Environment.   The nursing home environment offers a vast research arena to nurses interested in finding better ways to practice their art. Nurses and patients alike exist in this environment without thought of changing the physical setting to serve them better. For example, a major problem for many people is the need to adjust to a roommate. Nursing home policy is based on the interaction of residents when often the demand of nursing home residents is for privacy. Why, after 75 years of independent living, does the resident suddenly need to adjust to having a roommate?

Current bathing facilities is another area of concern. How many of us have participated in the shower ritual that takes place in the nursing home? The patients are naked and wheeled into a public shower area. The shower area is always cold and drafty, even on warm days. If the patients are fortunate enough to be draped, the drape is removed and the patients sit in their totality as they are scrubbed down in the presence of other naked patients. Three or four aides laugh and joke, while doing the job, and talk about their own trials and tribulations.

Kart (1981) described the above scene in its entirety, and likened the procedure to two sisters doing the dishes. The sisters, however, are more careful with the dishes than the aides might be with patients. Thus, the basic question for our environmental experts is, "How does one provide privacy and eliminate drafts in a shower room?" These questions demand the attention of researchers collaborating with architects, builders, and nurses in the planning stages of nursing home construction.

Perhaps brainstorming might answer some of these questions and provide new topics for study by researchers. For example, rather than large double rooms along a hallway, individual pods surrounding adequate bathing and toilet areas with communal but separate sitting rooms can be built. With such a model, patients will feel at home rather than in an institution. Each section can serve a different kind of resident, one for short-stay rehabilitation, and one for long-stay respite care. The sectioning also will assure that the nursing approach to the resident will be different as well. Figure 1 depicts this idea in part.

CONCLUSION

Nursing homes await appropriate research. They offer a stationary sample, simplifying the research process. The challenge for future research must be to improve the quality of life and the delivery of care in nursing homes, rather than just to study a captive sample.

Nursing home care belongs to nurses. Nurses make the decisions, provide the care, educate the caregivers, suggest changes, act as role models and influence the decisions of the physician. Nurses are responsible for the care that is delivered in nursing homes. Nurses should shoulder these responsibilities and use research in the institutional setting to model the highest quality of care in these complex

Figure 1

Modular Concept for Nursing Homes

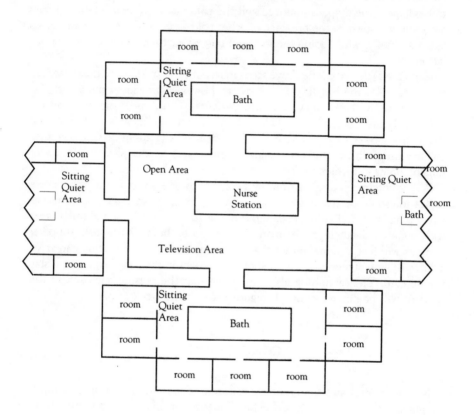

and differing patients. Nurse researchers have an opportunity to make a difference in the nursing home and they must rise to this challenge.

ACKNOWLEDGEMENTS

The author would like to thank Shirley Hendrix and George Campbell for their assistance in the preparation of this paper.

REFERENCES

Adams, F. (1988). Fluid intake: How much do elders drink? *Geriatric Nursing*, 9(4), 218–221.

Adams, F. (1988, July/August). *Geriatric Nursing*, 9(4).

Amenta, M., Weiner, A., & Amenta, D. (1984, November/December). Successful relocation. *Geriatric Nursing*, 5, 356–359.

Basson, P.H. (1967). The gerontological nursing literature search: Study and results. *Nursing Research*, 16, 267–272.

Benedict, S. (1975). *Medical care evaluation studies for utilization review in skilled nursing facilities*. Rockville, MD: Social Security Administration, Department of Health, Education, and Welfare).

Blom, M.F. (1985, March/April). Dramatic decrease in decubitus ulcers. *Geriatric Nursing*, 84–87.

Boykin, A., & Winland-Brown, J. (1986). Pressure sores: Nursing management. *Journal of Gerontological Nursing*, 12(12), 17–21.

Bristow, J.V., Goldfarb, E.H., & Green, M. (1987, May/June). Clinitron therapy: Is it effective? *Geriatric Nursing*, 120–124.

Burgio, L.D., Jones, L.T., Butler, F., & Engle, B.T. (1988). Behavior problems in an urban nursing home. *Journal of Gerontological Nursing*, 14(1), 31–34.

Burgio, L.D., Jones, L.T., & Engle, B.T., (1988). Studying incontinence in an urban nursing home. *Journal of Gerontological Nursing*, 14(4), 40–45.

Burnside, I. (1985). Gerontological nursing research: 1975 to 1984. In *Overcoming the bias of ageism in long-term care*. New York: National League for Nursing, pp. 121–138.

Diekmann, J.M. (1984). Use of a dental irrigation device in the treatment of decubitus ulcers. *Nursing Research*, 33(5), 303–305.

Doyle, G.C., Dunns, S.I., Thadani, I., & Lenihan, P. (1986). Investigating tools to aid in restorative care for Alzheimer's patients. *Journal of Gerontological Nursing*, 12(9), 19–24.

Eaton, M., Mitchell-Bonair, I.L., Friedmann, E., (1986). The effect of touch on nutritional intake of chronic organic brain syndrome patients. *Journal of Gerontology, 41*(5), 611–616.

Fakouri, C., & Jones, P. (1987). Relaxation RX: Slow stroke back rub. *Journal of Gerontological Nursing, 13*(2), 32–35.

Francis, G. & Baly, A. (1986, May/June). Plush animals— Do they make a difference? *Geriatric Nursing*, 140–142.

Gaspar, P.M. (1988). Fluid intake: What determines how much patients drink? *Geriatric Nursing, 9*(4), 221–224.

Gomez, G.E., Otto, D., Blattstein, A., & Gomez, E.A., (1985). Beginning nursing students can change attitudes about the aged. *Journal of Gerontological Nursing, 11*(1), 6–11.

Gunter, L.M., & Miller, J.C. (1977). Toward a nursing gerontology. *Nursing Research, 26*, 208–221.

Haeker, S. (1985, November/December). Disposable vs. reusable incontinence products. *Geriatric Nursing*, 345–347.

Heller, B.R., Bausell, R.B., & Ninos, M. (1984). Nurses' perceptions of rehabilitation potential of institutionalized aged. *Journal of Gerontological Nursing, 10*(7), 22–26.

Hollinger, L.M. (1986). Communicating with the elderly. *Journal of Gerontological Nursing, 12*(3), 9–13.

Hussian, R.A., & Brown, D.C., (1987). Use of two-dimensional grid patterns to limit hazardous ambulation in demented patients. *Journal of Gerontology, 42*(5), 558–560.

Kart, C.S. (1981). *The realities of aging: An introduction to gerontology.* Allyn and Bacon, Inc.

Kayser-Jones, J. (1981). Gerontological nursing research revisited. *Journal of Gerontological Nursing, 1*, 217–223.

Lappe, J.M. (1987). Reminiscing: The life review therapy. *Journal of Gerontological Nursing, 13*(4), 12–16.

Long, M.L., (1985). Incontinence. *Journal of Gerontological Nursing, 11*(1), 30–41.

Michaelsson, E., Norberg, A., & Norberg, B. (1987, March/April). Feeding methods for demented patients in end stage of life. *Geriatric Nursing*, 69–73.

Milton, I., & MacPhail, J. (1985, July/August). Dolls and toy animals for hospitalized elders—Infantilizing or comforting? *Geriatric Nursing*, 204–206.

Ouslander, J.G., Morishita, L., Blaustein, J., Orzeck, S., Dunn, S., & Sayre, J. (1987). Clinical, functional, and psychosocial characteristics of an incontinent nursing home population. *Journal of Gerontology, 42*(6), 631–637.

Pajk, M., Craven, G.A., Cameron, J., Shipps, T., & Bennum, N.W. (1986). Investigating the problem of pressure sores. *Gerontological Nursing, 12*(7), 11–16.

Pearson, B.D., & Droessler, D., Sr. (1988). Continence through nursing care. *Geriatric Nursing, 9*, 345–347.

Pensiero, M., & Adams, M. (1987). Dress and self-esteem. *Journal of Gerontological Nursing, 13*(10), 11–17.

Petrucci, K.E., McCormick K.A., & Scheve, A.A.S. (1987). Documenting patient care needs: Do nurses do it? *Journal of Gerontological Nursing, 13*(1), 34–38.

Pritchard, V. (1988). Tube feeding related pneumonias. *Journal of Gerontological Nursing, 14*(7), 32–36.

Reisberg, B. (1983). *Alzheimer's disease: The standard reference.* New York: The Free Press, Macmillan, Inc.

Roberts, B.L., & Lincoln, R.E. (1988). Cognitive disturbance in hospitalized and institutionalized elders. *Research in Nursing and Health, 11*(5), 309–319.

Robinson, L. (1981). Gerontological nursing Research. In I. Burnside (Ed.), *Nursing and the aged.* (2nd ed.). New York: McGraw-Hill, pp. 654–666.

Ryden, M.B. (1984). Morale and perceived control in institutionalized elderly. *Nursing Research, 33*(3), 130–136.

Ryden, M.B. (1985). Environmental support for autonomy in the institutionalized elderly. *Research in Nursing and Health, 8,* 363–371.

Slimmer, L.W., Lopez, M., LeSage, J., & Ellor, J.R. (1987). Perceptions of learned helplessness. *Journal of Gerontological Nursing, 13*(5), 33–37.

Sloane, P., Lekan-Rutledge, D., & Gilchrist, P. (1986). Telephone contacts in the decision-making process. *Journal of Gerontological Nursing, 12*(8), 35–39.

Spitzer, M.E. (1988). Taste acuity in institutionalized and non-institutionalized elderly men. *Journal of Gerontology, 43*(3), P71–P74.

Strumpf, N.E. (1986). Studying the language of time. *Journal of Gerontological Nursing, 12*(8), 22–26.

Stull, M.K., & Vernon, J.A. (1986). Nursing care needs are changing in facilities with rising patient acuity. *Journal of Gerontological Nursing, 12*(2), 15–19.

Travis, S. (1988). Observer-rated functional assessments for institutionalized elders. *Nursing Research, 37*(3), 138–143.

Whitman, S., & Kursh, E.D. (1987). Curbing incontinence. *Journal of Gerontological Nursing, 13*(4), 35–40.

Winger, J.M., & Smyth-Staruch, K. (1986). Your patient is older: What leads to job satisfaction? *Journal of Gerontological Nursing, 12*(1), 31–35.

Wirtz, B.J. (1987). Effects of air and water mattresses on thermoregulation. *Journal of Gerontological Nursing, 13*(5), 13–17.

Yu, L. (1987). Incontinence stress index: Measuring psychological impact. *Journal of Gerontological Nursing, 13*(7), 18–25.

Yu, L.C., & Kaltreider, D.L. (1987). Stressed nurses: Dealing with incontinent patients. *Journal of Gerontological Nursing, 13*(1), 27–30.

Appendix I
Long-Term Care

Other

Author	Journal	Purpose
Alvarez, S., Shell, C.G., Woolley, T.W., Berk, S.L., & Smith, J.K.	*Journal of Gerontology*, (1988). Nosocomial Infections in Long-Term Facilities. 43(1), M9–M15.	To determine incidence and prevalence of nosocomial infections in skilled nursing care and nursing home units and identify risk factors.
Kim, K.K.	*Research in Nursing and Health*, (1986). Response Time and Health Care Learning of Elderly Patients. Vol 9, 233–239.	Do elderly patients perform better in health care learning when provided slower or self-paced response conditions.
Pensiero, M., & Adams, M.	*Journal of Gerontological Nursing*, (1987). Dress and Self-Esteem. 13(10), 11–17.	Examine association between dress and self-esteem.
Petrucci, K.E., McCormick, K.A., & Scheve, A.A.S.	*Journal of Gerontological Nursing*, (1987). Documenting Patient Care Needs: Do Nurses Do It? 13(11), 34–38.	Examine nurses documentation of patient care needs.
Pritchard, V.	*Journal of Gerontological Nursing*, (1988). Tube Feeding Related Pneumonias. 14(7), 32–36.	Discover if new small-bore tubes result in fewer nasogastric tube-related infections and so are safer.
Ryden, M.B.	*Nursing Research*, (1984). Morale and Perceived Control in Institutionalized Elderly. 33(3), 130–136.	To explore patterns of causal relationship of situational control, health, socioeconomic status, functional dependency, length of stay, and morale in institutionalized elderly.

Other

#	Design	Results	AP
132	4-year routine surveillance of nosocomial infections. Last year, one day/month visit of infection control team. N = 132 males, mean age = 68.2, divided into 3 wards.	Wide variations in hospital acquired infections in long-term care depends on level of care required by patient. Nosocomial infections are common among residents in long-term care facilities.	no
105	After nutrition instruction learning performance measured.	A self-paced response condition is advantageous for elderly patients.	yes
40	Compare groups from 2 nursing homes. 30 interviews of 5-minute duration over 5-week period.	Residents in dress had increased self-esteem and were more independent.	yes
162	Retrospective descriptive chart audit.	Documentation varied according to the tools used. Weekly nurse summary.	no
42	20 tube feedings via small-bore feeding tubes, 22 tube feedings via large-bore Levine type tubes.	4 small bore patients developed pneumonia, 20%. 12 Levine-type patients developed pneumonia, 54.5%. Small bore tubes associated with fever URI, fewer pneumonia, and fewer instances of tube displacement or aspiration.	yes
133	From 4 nursing homes, intermediate and skilled care wards. Age above 60, mean age = 80.9. Variables determined with interviews and measurement tools. Patients had auditory, acuity, and cognitive competence. Patients selected by investigator. Mean length of stay 34.1 months for residents on intermediate care and 30.8 months for residents on skilled care.	Perception of situational control was a key variable, significantly related to morale of patients on skilled care wards. Greater the functional dependency, less sense of control and lower morale score. Length of institutionalization had no effect.	yes

Other (Continued)

Author	Journal	Purpose
Ryden, M.B.	*Research in Nursing and Health,* (1985). Environmental Support for Autonomy in the Institutionalized Elderly. Vol 8, 363–371.	Part of larger study of relationship between perception of situational control and morale. This explores aspects of nursing home environment that influences potential for degree of autonomy of residents.
Sloane, P., Lekan-Rutledge, D., & Gilchrist, P.	*Journal of Gerontological Nursing,* (1986). Telephone Contacts in the Decision-Making Process. *12*(8), 35–39.	Descriptive study to understand better use of telephone contact in decision making in a nursing home.
Strumpf, N.E.	*Journal of Gerontological Nursing,* (1986). Studying the Language of Time. *12*(8), 22–26.	Identify differences in time experience among those in independent, intermediate, and skilled nursing units, and examine responses for meaning of time among elderly in nursing home settings.
Stull, M.K., & Vernon, J.A.	*Journal of Gerontological Nursing,* (1986). Nursing Care Needs Are Changing in Facilities With Rising Patient Acuity. *12*(2), 15–19.	Explore recent increase of acuity level in long-term care facility.
Wirtz, B.J.	*Journal of Gerontological Nursing,* (1987). Effects of Air and Water Mattresses on Thermoregulation. *13*(5), 13–17.	Determine if patients on unheated water mattress have a lower body temperature than those on an alternating air mattress.

Other (Continued)

#	Design	Results	AP
250	N = 113, 54 skilled care, 59 intermediate care. N = 137 caregivers. Two questionnaires administered to staff and two questionnaires administered to residents.	Residents and caregivers similar in perceptions of power of residents. 70% of administration thought residents had less power.	no
637	2 nursing homes, (1) 60 skilled-care beds, (2) 60 skilled-care and 58 intermediate. Care data collected on records for each series of communications on one patient = one contact.	637 contacts, 81% generated physician orders. 29% represented drug prescriptions, 71% related to identified clinical problems. Critical decisions are frequently made by telephone and physicians made medical decisions based on nurse assessments.	
50	Volunteers from long-term care unit. Individual interviews and testing. 17 from independent living. 17 from intermediate care. 16 from skilled care.	Not easily quantified. Independent living—aware of changing relationships of time. Intermediate care—struggling with growing dependency. Skilled care—accepting the end of life.	no
25	Survey 1 group with questionnaire.	96% said increased acuity level. Impact on nurse workload staff development programs, staffing patterns, and organizational policies and practices.	yes
20	Conceptional random selection descriptive study. Over age 62, 72-hour period.	Patients on water mattresses have lower skin temperature and lower sublingual temperature.	yes

Incontinence

Author	Journal	Purpose
Burgio, L.D., Jones, L.T., & Engle, B.T.	*Journal of Gerontological Nursing*, (1988). Studying Incontinence in an Urban Nursing Home. *14*(4), 40–45.	To examine intensively continent and incontinent geriatric nursing home patients on a number of dimensions including mobility, toileting, functional deficits, behavior excesses, medical condition, and medication.
Haeker, S.	*Geriatric Nursing*, (1985). Disposable vs. Reusable Incontinence Products. Nov/Dec, 345–347.	Test disposable vs. washable incontinence-care undergarment.
Long, M.L.	*Journal of Gerontological Nursing*, (1985). *11*(1), 30–41.	Determine incidence of urinary incontinence and demonstrate results of nursing intervention.
Ouslander, J.G., Morishita, L., Blaustein, J., Orzeck, S., Dunn, S., & Sayre, J.	*Journal of Gerontology*, (1987). Clinical, Functional, and Psychosocial Characteristics of an Incontinent Nursing Home Population. *42*(6), 631–637.	To compare clinical, functional, and psychosocial characteristics of continent and incontinent nursing home residents.
Pearson, B.D., & Droessler, D., Sr.	*Geriatric Nursing*, (1988). Continence Through Nursing Care. 9(6), 347–349.	To investigate effectiveness of noninvasive strategies used to diagnose and treat actual and potential loss of urine control in elderly.
Whitman, S., & Kursh, E.D.	*Journal of Gerontological Nursing*, (1987). Curbing Incontinence. *13*(4), 35–40.	Show that medical and nursing interventions improve incontinence.
Yu, L.	*Journal of Gerontological Nursing*, (1987). Incontinence Stress Index: Measuring Psychological Impact. *13*(7), 18–25.	Development of patient Incontinence Stress Index.
Yu, L.C., & Kaltreider, D.L.	*Journal of Gerontological Nursing*, (1987). Stressed Nurses: Dealing With Incontinent Patients. *13*(1), 27–30.	Explore staff stress caused by incontinent patients.

Incontinence

#	Design	Results	AP
154	45-minute interview with nursing assistants on patients' mobility, continence, abilities, behavioral deficits, and excesses. Review of medical records.	54% incontinent patients displayed impairments in cognition and mobility. 41% of mobility impairment patients had cognitive deficit. 29% of continent patients had significant cognitive and mobility impairments.	yes
26	Clinical trial of 2 groups. 3-week trial.	8% had skin problems pretrial. 22% during trial. Disposable product unsatisfactory.	yes
14	Assess patients admitted to 15 bed geriatric unit; 75 > older and retrain those at risk for 7 months.	11 of 14 successful. 10 of 11 successful but require some assistance or reminder.	yes no
100	50 = continent 50 = incontinent. Assessments, medical reviews, urinalysis and culture, timed test of skills were examined related to toileting.	Association between functional disability and incontinence. No difference in morale status of two groups. Significant bacteriuria more common in incontinent group. Incontinent patients did not differ significantly from continent on measures of social and recreational activities except for less agile.	
74	All at risk or incontinent. Room and board facility and infirmary of 22 beds. Histories of urinary incontinence, monthly for 6 months pretreatment. Treatment = noninvasive strategies started first month.	6 reversals of incontinence. All 74 significantly decreased number of risk indicators experienced. Liquid intake increased for older elderly by 250cc daily.	yes
8	One group intervention descriptive.	6 of 8 improved with therapy; 50 percent had URI; 5 of 8 had neurogenic bladder.	yes
27	12 in control group, 15 in experimental group plus 3 who did not participate in training. Majority over age 75. Only newly diagnosed incontinent and newly admitted incontinent.	Urinary incontinence is stressful for patients.	yes
156	Convenience sample, survey questionnaire, 30 items.	Staff experienced psychological stress in connection with incontinence.	no

25

Food and Fluids

Author	Journal	Purpose
Adams, F.	*Geriatric Nursing*, (1988). Fluid Intake: How Much Do Elders Drink? 9(4), 218–221.	To describe and compare fluid intake practices of institutionalized and non-institutionalized elderly in relation to time pattern, amount, and type of fluid intake.
Eaton, M., Mitchell-Bonair, I.L., & Friedmann, E.	*Journal of Gerontology*, (1986). The Effect of Touch on Nutritional Intake of Chronic Organic Brain Syndrome Patients, 41(5), 611–616.	To study effects of gentle touch with oral encouragement to promote self-feeding and improve nutritional intake of chronic organic brain syndrome patients in institutions.
Gaspar, P.M.	*Geriatric Nursing*, (1988). Fluid Intake: What Determines How Much Patients Drink? 9(4), 221–224.	Document determinants of adequate and inadequate patient water intake.
Michaelsson, E., Norberg, A., & Norberg, B.	*Geriatric Nursing*, (1987). Feeding Methods for Demented Patients in End-Stage of Life. Mar/Apr, 69–73.	Describe eating difficulties of patients with senile dementia.
Spitzer, M.E.	*Journal of Gerontology*, (1988). Taste Acuity in Institutionalized and Noninstitutionalized Elderly Men. 43(3), P71–P74.	To examine taste ability in institutionalized elderly by comparing to noninstitutionalized elderly adults and young adults.

Foods and Fluids

#	Design	Results	AP
60	30 = institutionalized, 30 = noninstitutionalized. Age = 65 > 85. Those with cognitive impairment, major disabilities, and diabetes mellitus excluded. Three different long-term care facilities, questionnaire for status. Instructed for 3 days on fluid intake measuring and recording. Records collected.	Both groups had 75% of fluid intake between 6 AM and 6 PM. Institutionalized met norm for adult intake. Noninstitutionalized exceeded norm. Institutionalized had intake at mealtime and medicine time.	yes
42	21 = control group, 21 = experimental group. Skilled care facility. Control group mean age = 85.4 with mean length of stay = 35.9 months. Single investigator observed food intake of each person over 3, 5-day weeks. 1st 5 days = baseline 2nd 5 days = treatment 3rd 5 days = posttreatment, touch treatment.	Touch had a significant positive effect on nutritional intake of chronic organic brain syndrome patients.	yes
67	2 rural nursing homes. Convenience sample observational design.	Intake inadequate: variables: age, functional and speaking ability.	yes
400	Observation, some structured interviews.	69 severe eating difficulties. 4 common problem eating-behaviors, most could be spoon feed.	yes
47	All men. Control young group. N=15, mean age = 21.4. Noninstitutionalized elderly N=17, mean age = 73.2. Institutionalized elderly N=15, mean age = 74.6. Biographical questionnaire with disease status and medications. Taste testing under controlled situation.	Results suggest detection thesis holds for sour and salt. Bitter increased with age. Sweet unrelated to age. Significant difference for institutionalized on medication to sour with increased sour detection threshold. Hypertensive patients on medication had significant increase in salt threshold.	no

Pressure Sores

Author	Journal	Purpose
Blom, M.F.	*Geriatric Nursing*, (1985). Dramatic Decrease in Decubitus Ulcers. Mar/Apr, 84–87.	3-year assessment of decubiti and collection of data on treatment.
Boykin, A., & Winland-Brown, J.	*Journal of Gerontological Nursing*, (1986). Pressure Sores: Nursing Management. 12(12), 17–21.	Evaluate if adherence to prescribed prevention guidelines, for clients determined at risk, resulted in improvement in risk status. Compare effectiveness of hydrocolloid occlusive dressing, with povidone-iodine therapy in treatment of pressure sores.
Bristow, J.V., Goldfarb, E.H., & Green, M.	*Geriatric Nursing*, (1987). Clinitron Therapy: Is it Effective? May/Jun, 120–124.	Examine Clinitron bed for decubiti care.
Diekmann, J.M.	*Nursing Research*, (1984). Use of a Dental Irrigating Device in the Treatment of Decubitus Ulcers. 33(5), 303–305.	To determine if dental irrigating device could be successfully employed to treat decubitus ulcer with saline.
Pajk, M., Craven, G.A., Cameron, J., Shipps, T., & Bennum, N.W.	*Journal of Gerontological Nursing*, (1986). Investigating the Problem of Pressure Sores. 12(7), 11–16.	Identify patients at risk for development of pressure sores.

Pressure Sores

#	Design	Results	AP
27	Quality assurance data.	81.5% overall reduction rate of decubitus ulcer, but no one medical treatment, nursing measure, or device determined to be effective for all patients.	yes
21	Mean age = 83, range 67–96. All in home health care. 11 had pressure sores, 10 were at risk, but without pressure sores for 1 to 12 weeks. Norton scale for potentiality. Families and patients given oral and written instructions. Weekly visit. All participated in first hypothesis; 11 pressure sores treated with povidone-iodine. 10 pressure sores treated with hydrocolloid occlusive dressing.	Pressure sores treated with hydrocolloid occlusive dressing showed decrease in size twice that of povidone-iodine. Did not support hypothesis of significant change in at risk adhering to prevention guidelines.	yes yes
10	Observation of intervention convenience sample.	Clinitron bed highly effective in healing decubiti.	yes
16	Mean age = 83.6, range 55–96. Tracing done of ulcers pre/post-test, 1 group of 8 treated with saline irrigation 2 x daily x 2 weeks, no dressings used. 1 group of 8 given only routine care as normally provided.	In both groups all but 3 ulcers decreased in size. No support for use of irrigation device in treatment.	
208	Audit of 10 units for 10 days using assessment tools of Gornell and Norton for risk factors and skin integrity.	Substantiate clinical relevance of using risk factor identification tool.	yes

Nursing Intervention

Author	Journal	Purpose
Eaton, M., Mitchell-Bonair, I.L., & Friedmann, E.	*Journal of Gerontology*, (1986). The Effect of Touch on Nutritional Intake of Chronic Brain Syndrome Patients. *41*(5), 611–616.	To study effects of gentle touch with oral encouragement to promote self-feeding and improve nutritional intake of chronic organic brain syndrome patients in institutions.
Fakouri, C., & Jones, P.	*Journal of Gerontological Nursing*, (1987). Relaxation RX; Slow Stroke Back Rub. *13*(2), 32–35.	Test slow stroke back rub as a relaxation promoting measure.
Francis, G., & Baly, A.	*Geriatric Nursing*, (1986). Plush Animals—Do They Make A Difference? May/Jun, 140–142.	Do plush animals make a difference?
Hollinger, L.M.	*Journal of Gerontological Nursing*, (1986). Communicating with the Elderly. *12*(3), 9–13.	Is there a relationship between nurse touch and length and frequency of oral response by elderly.
Lappe, J.M.	*Journal of Gerontological Nursing*, (1987). Reminiscing: The Life Review Therapy. *13*(4), 12–16.	Compare reminiscing group to other type group; met 10 weeks.
Milton, I., & MacPhail, J.	*Geriatric Nursing*, (1985). Dolls and Toy Animals for Hospitalized Elders—Infantilizing or Comforting? Jul/Aug, 204–206.	Investigate use of stuffed animals.

Nursing Intervention

#	Design	Results	AP
42	21 = control group, 21 = experimental group. Skilled care facility. Control group mean age = 85.4 with mean length of stay = 35.9 months. Single investigator observed food intake of each person over 3, 5-day weeks. 1st 5 days = baseline 2nd 5 days = treatment 3rd 5 days = posttreatment, touch treatment.	Touch had a significant positive effect on nutritional intake of chronic organic brain syndrome patients.	yes
18	One experimental group. Pre- and posttested. Average age = 73.7.	Produced findings that suggest it produces a relaxation response in elderly clients.	yes
40	Pre- and posttesting with experimental and control groups.	Introduction of plush animals made a significant, positive difference in multiple psychosocial aspects.	yes
8	Experimental with partial counter balancing.	Duration of oral responses increased with touch, frequency of oral responses increased with nurse touch.	yes
83	Control and experimental groups with pretest, posttest. 10 weeks.	Reminiscing increased self-esteem, but group meeting 2 x week did not show statistical difference from group meeting once-a-week.	yes
10	Elderly and families. Survey, oral and observational.	Not infantilism.	yes

Behavior

Author	Journal	Purpose
Bernier, S.L., & Small, N.R.	*Journal of Gerontological Nursing*, (1988). Disruptive Behaviors. *14*(2), 8–13.	To describe specific disruptive behaviors of residents.
Burgio, L.D., Jones, L.T., Butler, F., & Engle, B.T.	*Journal of Gerontological Nursing*, (1988). Behavior Problems in an Urban Nursing Home. *14*(1), 31–34.	To intensively examine all intermediate and skilled care patients in nursing homes for occurrence of significant behavior problems.
Roberts, B.L., & Lincoln, R.E.	*Research in Nursing and Health*, (1988). Cognitive Disturbance in Hospitalized and Institutionalized Elders. *11*(5), 309–319.	Examine variables causing cognitive disturbance in hospitals and institutions.
Slimmer, L.W., Lopez, M., LeSage, J., & Ellor, J.R.	*Journal of Gerontological Nursing*, (1987). Perceptions of Learned Helplessness. *13*(5), 33–37.	To describe nurses' perceptions of learned helplessness. Separate adoptive behaviors from learned helplessness behaviors.

Behavior

#	Design	Results	AP
110	Residents N = 44, Nursing Staff = 66. Questionnaires of both groups—job satisfaction questionnaire to staff. Residents interviewed individually.	No commonality of items between staff and residents suggest need to look at differences, perception, and understanding of terminology.	yes
160	Behavior problems survey assessment tool administered to 35 nursing staff on 160 patients.	Behavior problems occur at rates which are clinically significant in a geriatric long-term care setting.	yes
172	Random sample of patients over 65 years of age. 94 in acute-care facility. 78 long-term nursing care. These 2 groups compared with examinations, questionnaires, medical record review.	Neuronal function associated with cognitive loss. Sensory deficit problem in hospital environment and probably in nursing homes.	yes
28 RN	Qualitative descriptive. Voluntary participation.	RN viewed qualitative learned helplessness as undesirable. 13 stated learned helplessness was way of decreasing loneliness, getting attention, or controlling staff and circumstances. 11 said from fear, negative attitude. 5 said due to family's reinforcement.	no

33

Communication and Interaction

Author	Journal	Purpose
Huss, M.J., Buckwalter, K.C., & Stolley, J.	*Journal of Gerontological Nursing*, (1988). Nursing Impact on Life Satisfaction. *14*(5), 31–36.	To identify the association between life satisfaction and perception of the nurse/resident relationship.
Loveridge, C.E., & Heineken, J.	*Journal of Gerontological Nursing*, (1988). Confirming Interactions. *14*(5), 27–30.	To show a reciprocal relationship of confirming/disconfirming communication patterns and to show relationship between job satisfaction and quality care.
Wagnild, G., & Manning, R.W.	*Journal of Gerontological Nursing*, (1985). Convey Respect During Bathing Procedures (Patient Well-Being Depends On It!). *11*(12), 6–10.	Observe interaction between resident and nurse aide during bath.
Doyle, G.C., Dunn, S.I., Thadani, I., & Lenihan, P.	*Journal of Gerontological Nursing*, (1986). Investigating Tools to Aid in Restorative Care for Alzheimer's Patients. *12*(9), 19–24.	Study of standardized assessment tools to measure capability of individuals with Alzheimer's disease.
Engle, V.F., Wahl, A., Dimond, C., & Bobel, L.	*Journal of Gerontological Nursing*, (1985). Tardive Dyskinesia: Are Your Older Clients at Risk? *11*(9), 25–37.	Examine impact of tardive dyskinesia on activities of daily living. Which activities most impaired.
Golander, H.	*Journal of Gerontological Nursing*, (1987). Under the Guise of Passivity. *13*(2), 26–31.	Reveal the active role of the disabled in shaping their lives in institutional settings.
Helmes, E., Csapo, K.G., & Short, J.A.	*Journal of Gerontology*, (1987). Standardization and Validation of the Multi-Dimensional Observation Scale for Elderly Subjects (MOSES). *42*(4), 395–405.	Effectiveness of Multidimensional Observation Scale for Elderly Subjects to provide reliable valid staff ratings of major areas of clinical concern to health care staff.

Communication and Interaction

#	Design	Results	AP
30	Mean age = 85. 6-part interview of residents. Barthal Index, Individual Perception of Health Status, HRCA Social Contact Inventory, 3rd area of Risser Tool, Life Satisfaction Index, and demographic data for profile of sample.	Nurse/resident relationship did not correlate significantly with life satisfaction. Health status perception had highest impact on life satisfaction.	no
300	300 bed long-term care institution. Questionnaires and observations by skilled research assistant.	Confirming/disconfirming communication framework not significant. Correlation between job satisfaction and "quality care" was supported.	yes
42	1 observed group with questionnaire and observation checklist.	50% of residents engaged in conversation, 33% prepared. Need to make bath quality time.	yes
25	Mean age = 80.6. Assessed with CADET and FROMAJE—patients on skilled nursing facility, Alzheimer's unit.	Findings can't be generalized until more formal study is done.	yes
60	1 group random selection given activities of Daily Living Index.	Relationship identified between tardive dyskinesia symptoms and difficulty in performing everyday tasks.	no
43	Anthropologic field work, 1 year (500 hours) to cover 24 hours of day, weekdays, and weekend observations.	Just coping with simple daily activities demands much persistence, patience, strength, and ingenuity.	no
*	* = 2,542. Ratings of institutionalized elderly. 151 below age 65, mean age = 81. 7 psychiatric facilities, 22 nursing homes, 9 homes for aged, 7 continuing care hospitals. Instructions to nursing staffs. All raters had daily contact with individuals studied.	In general, Multidimensional Observation Scale for Elderly Subjects shows satisfactory interrater reliability. Offers several specific advantages over other scales. Shows promise as an assessment tool for institutionalized elderly.	yes

Communication and Interaction (Continued)

Author	Journal	Purpose
Pruchno, R.A., Kleban, M.H., & Resch, N.L.	*Journal of Gerontology*, (1988). Psychometric Assessment of the Multidimensional Observation Scale for Elderly Subjects (MOSES). *43*(6), P164–P168.	Study usefulness of revised Multidimensional Observation Scale for Elderly Subjects as research and clinical tool.
Travis, S.	*Nursing Research*, (1988). Observer-Rated Functional Assessments for Institutionalized Elders. *37*(3), 138–143.	Assess function through observation and content analysis.

#	Design	Results	AP
536	Residents of Jewish Home for Aged. Behavioral observations using Multidimensional Observation Scale for Elderly Subjects. 36 nursing assistants instructed in purpose and importance of observation. Mean age = 86.3.	Revised Multidimensional Observation Scale for Elderly Subjects offers advantages over other instruments to measure behaviors of institutionalized elderly.	yes
40	Observational data on functional behaviors of institutionalized psychogeriatric patients and content analysis.	Identified 3 behavioral constructs that correlated somewhat with behaviors on existing scales and identify Moses as most complete observer-rated functional assessment tool.	yes

Falls

Author	Journal	Purpose
Daley, I., & Goldman, L.	*Geriatric Nursing*, (1987). A Closer Look At Institutional Accidents. Mar/Apr, 64–67.	Identify patterns and causes of patients' accidents and incidents. Develop criteria for identifying those at high risk and improve nurse accountability to develop strategies for accident prevention.
Hernandez, M., & Miller, J.	*Geriatric Nursing*, (1986). How to Reduce Falls. Mar/Apr, 97–102.	Intervention study to reduce falls.
Venglarik, J.M., & Adams, M.	*Journal of Gerontological Nursing*, (1985). Which Client is a High Risk? *11*(5), 28–30.	3-year study of incidence, circumstance, and resultant injuries with nursing home residents, due to falls.

Falls

#	Design	Results	AP
88	88 bed skilled-care facility in 2-year study. Observations of first year changes made. Observed second year.	Focusing on nurse accountability in accident prevention had significant impact on reducing accident rate 2nd year.	yes
108	One group observational report.	Define risk factors and put prevention program in process. Falls decreased.	yes
221	Chart scan of all residents.	221 residents involved in 933 reported falls. 59% on skilled nursing floors. 88.7% women. 68.8% fell more than once. 40.3% in bed room and in single rooms. 30% minor injuries. 42% on day-shift.	yes

Relocation

Author	Journal	Purpose
Amenta, M., Weiner, A., & Amenta, D.	*Geriatric Nursing*, (1984). Successful Relocation, Nov/Dec, Vol 5, 356–359.	Study effects of deliberate choice making in forced relocation of elderly institutionalized.
Engle, V.F.	*Research in Nursing and Health*, (1985). Mental Status and Functional Health Following Relocation to a Nursing Home. Vol 8, 355–361.	Measure stability of mental status and functional health immediately following relocation from hospital to nursing home.
Engle, V.F.	*Journal of Gerontological Nursing*, (1985). Temporary Relocation: Is It Stressful to Your Patients? 11(10), 28–31.	Study stability of mental status and activities of daily living during first week of nursing home admission.
Pearlman, R.A., & Ryan-Dykes, M.	*Journal of Gerontological Nursing*, (1986). The Vulnerable Elderly. 12(9), 15–18.	Identify predictors of nursing home placement among vulnerable elderly population.

Relocation

#	Design	Results	AP
70	N = 47 forced relocations, mean age 75. Stay at previous facility 1 to 24 years. Pre-move studies and post-move tests. 12 = residents who chose to relocate within new facility, mean age = 80. 11 = refused to relocate in new facility, mean age = 85. Total N = 70.	No increase for death rate of any group in 6 months post-move. Forced transfer group showed marked decrease in death rate. All groups deteriorated over 6-month period but stationary group showed greatest deterioration. Relocation had some life enhancing effects.	yes
55	Mental status exam, interview, and testing by same interviewer after first full day of admission and after fourth full day.	No significant difference on mental status. Functional ability increased slightly in all areas except feeding ability, and bladder and bowel continence.	yes
57	Average age = 80.5. One group. Questionnaires, 2 interviews first and seventh day of admission.	Mental status and function improved and stabilized during first week following admission.	yes
255	Median age = 78. Secondary data analysis of the Older American's Resources and Services (OARS) questionnaire used in demonstration project for prospective identification.	5 questions in OARS were predictive of nursing home placement. Other questions showing change within 6 months also predictive. Use predictors and plan.	yes

Attitude

Author	Journal	Purpose
Gomez, G.E., Otto, D., Blattstein, A., & Gomez, E.A.	*Journal of Gerontological Nursing*, (1985). Beginning Nursing Students Can Change Attitudes About the Aged. *11*(1), 6–11.	Investigate attitudes of RNs in 3-week course in nursing home.
Heller, B.R., Bausell, R.B., & Ninos, M.	*Journal of Gerontological Nursing*, (1984). Nurses' Perceptions of Rehabilitation Potential of Institutionalized Aged. *10*(7), 22–26.	To determine relationships between nurses perceptions of goals of institutional care and attitudes toward elderly.
Winger, J.M., & Smyth-Staruch, K.	*Journal of Gerontological Nursing*, (1986). Your Patient is Older: What Leads to Job Satisfaction? *12*(1), 31–35.	Delineate nurse attitude toward elderly patient.

Attitude

#	Design	Results	AP
82	One group survey questionnaire, Kogan's.	Significant increase in positive attitude toward the elderly.	yes
183	183 of 303 invited nurses (practical and registered) responded from 3 nursing homes. 59% registered nurses, 41% practical nurses. Demographic variables ascertained; questions administered and questionnaires statistically evaluated.	Significant relationship between attitudes and perceptions of care. Negative attitudes = more perceived custodial care. Positive attitudes = more rehabilitative orientation.	yes
±300	New questionnaire. Distributed to RNs on duty in a 4-day period. Approximately 300 nurses on duty in this period.	202, 67% returned. Decreased knowledge of geriatrics correlated with decreased desire to care for elderly. Increased knowledge does not influence desire to work.	yes

Confusion

Author	Journal	Purpose
Brady, P.F.	*Journal of Gerontological Nursing, (1987). Labeling of Confusion in the Elderly.* 13(6), 29–32.	Examine behaviors that label confusion.
Lincoln, R.	*Journal of Gerontological Nursing, (1984). What Do Nurses Know About Confusion in the Aged?* 10(8), 26–32.	Assess level of knowledge and opinions of nursing staff about reversible and irreversible forms of confusion.

Confusion

#	Design	Results	AP
25	Descriptive relationship between behaviors and confusion.	Time dissonant, disorientation to place and people, and hallucinations. Regardless of staff position, there is minimal ability to identify confusion.	yes
110	75 licensed and 35 unlicensed nursing personnel. 2 philanthropic nursing homes, 3-part investigator designed instrument questionnaire.	Subjects had considerable knowledge of reversible and irreversible confusion. Older and less educated had lower knowledge scores. Total sample had increased percent of incorrect responses in areas of irreversible sources of confusion.	yes

Sleep

Author	Journal	Purpose
Bahr, R.T., & Gress, L.	*Journal of Gerontological Nursing*, (1985). The 24-Hour Cycle: Rhythms of Health Sleep (Developing Nursing Strategies). *11*(4), 14–17.	Determine time increment of phases of sleep/wakefulness in 24-hour cycle.
Johnson, J.	*Journal of Gerontological Nursing*, (1985). Drug Treatment for Sleep Disturbances: Does It Really Work? *11*(8), 8–12.	Study the effect of narcoleptics on nocturnal sleep patterns and daytime behaviors.

Sleep

#	Design	Results	AP
12	Observation of convenience sample for 3, 24-hour days awake and asleep.	Baseline info on sleep/wake patterns of institutionalized adults. Variability.	yes
75	24 administered acetaminophen, 26 administered benzodiazepine, 25 no medication.	Benzodiazepines taken over 30 days showed significant changes. Prolonged sleep onset latencies, more frequent awaking and dissatisfied with sleep.	yes

Drugs

Author	Journal	Purpose
Butler, F.R., Burgio, L.D., & Engle, B.T.	*Journal of Gerontological Nursing*, (1987). Neuroleptics and Behavior: A Comparative Study. *13*(6), 15–19.	Examine the impact of neuroleptic medicine on behavior.
Thomas, B., & Price, M.	*Journal of Gerontological Nursing*, (1987). Drug Reviews. *13*(4), 17–21.	Describe Medicare drug reviews.

Drugs

#	Design	Results	AP
48	Convenience sample with random assignment ex post facto.	No definite activities of daily living falls, increased behavior problems, decreased grip strength, and increased physical problems.	yes
186	Survey. 284 questionnaires sent. 186 usable responses.	84% conduct monthly drug review. Drug irregularities identified in order of frequency. Laboratory tests needed. Lack of re-evaluation of drug orders. Many drug interactions and outdated drug orders.	no

Alzheimer's Disease

Author	Journal	Purpose
Doyle, G.C., Dunn, S.I., Thadani, I., & Lenihan, P.	*Journal of Gerontological Nursing*, (1986). Investigating Tools to Aid in Restorative Care for Alzheimer's Patients. *12*(9), 19–24.	Study of standardized assessment tools to measure capability of individuals with Alzheimer's disease.
Hussian, R.A., & Brown, D.C.	*Journal of Gerontology*, (1987). Use of Two-Dimensional Grid Patterns to Limit Hazardous Ambulation in Demented Patients. *42*(5), 558–560.	Study perception of visual stimulus as preventive barrier to prevent wandering by Alzheimer's patients.

Alzheimer's Disease

#	Design	Results	AP
25	Mean age = 80.6. Patients in skilled nursing facility on Alzheimer's unit assessed with Communication, Ambulation, Daily Activities, Elimination and Transfer (CADET) and Function, Reason, Orientation, Memory, Arithmetic, Judgment, and Emotional Status (FROMAJE) self-care and mental status evaluation tools.	Findings can't be generalized until more formal study is done.	yes
8	All males, mean age = 78.5. All ambulatory. Baseline study of ambulation pretest. Various grid patterns of tape on floor. Observation.	7 of 8 patients showed decreases in ambulation to exit doors. One pattern was more effective in preventing most patient exits.	yes

3

Response to: "Research in Long-Term Care: 1984-1988"

Sister Rose Therese Bahr, PhD, RN, FAAN
Professor of Nursing
Chair, Division of Community Health Nursing
The Catholic University of America School of Nursing
Washington, DC

In the minds of researchers, members of the scientific community, and legislators who seek data to promote improvement of health care delivery, nursing's claim to professionalism is growing stronger. As a result, the National Center for Nursing Research, American Nurses' Foundation, and private funding sources are providing more funds for research. Graduate programs in nursing are advocating that research is key for the improvement of nursing care in the clinical settings in which nurses practice. The importance of research also is stressed as one of the main objectives of the National League for Nursing Long-Term Care Committee of which this author is a member. As a colleague nurse educator and researcher, it is a privilege, therefore, to present a response to the overview of gerontologic nursing research conducted in long-term care settings for the years, 1984–1988, by Dr. Barbara Haight, Associate Professor of Nursing and Project Director of a federally funded Graduate Program in Gerontological Nursing, Medical University of South Carolina.

Because of its scholarly nature and comprehensive approach to research relevant to long-term care settings, Dr. Haight's paper was a pleasure to review.

Commendation is given to the author for a thorough, thoughtful, and provocative exposé of the state-of-the-art in nursing research in gerontological nursing. This realistic portrayal of the data, its analysis and implications for gerontological nursing, brings to the foreground the urgent necessity for encouragement of more research to promote the well-being of older adults residing in long-term care facilities. In such settings, older adults are dependent upon knowledgeable, skillful nurses who are current in their practice based on relevant research findings.

My response identifies the strengths and weaknesses of the four areas of research literature reviewed and discussed by Dr. Haight. Each area is examined and, where appropriate, problems/concerns are raised to emphasize the difficulties within the field of gerontological nursing research. The four areas or organizing themes of Haight's paper include: (1) past reviews of gerontological nursing research; (2) findings from a current search of nursing research in long-term care facilities; (3) current trends; and (4) suggestions for future research.

PAST REVIEWS OF GERONTOLOGICAL NURSING RESEARCH

Dr. Haight carefully reviewed literature identifying past reviews of a similar nature conducted by Basson (1967), Gunter and Miller (1977), Robinson (1981), and Kayser-Jones (1981). Each of these reviews noted particular deficiencies in the area of research in gerontological nursing. Haight based the foundation for her paper on the assessment of gerontological nursing research accomplished by Burnside (1985), which provides a complete overview of nursing research with a specific focus on long-term care. The strength of this paper, therefore, resides in the building up of areas that have been researched and a listing of the deficiencies or areas still needing to be researched. Unfortunately, the latter 28 research areas identified by Burnside have still not been undertaken in studies, demonstrating a lack of major attention to upgrading the clinical knowledge and nursing care of older residents particularly in long-term care facilities. This spanning of 20 years for gerontological nursing research demonstrates the scantiness of research studies and the infancy of the field with its contributions to a definitive body of knowledge for application in clinical settings.

Specifically, Haight noted deficiencies in these realms: the absence of theoretical frameworks and the use of rigid research designs; major emphasis on study of nurse attitudes and psychosocial needs of patients with little study on physical needs of patients; no longitudinal studies; and, no health promotion and disease prevention studies. Clearly, there currently is a fragmentation of research studies conducted in long-term care facilities. Consequently, a major concern in gerontological nursing research is the phenomenon of one-time studies conducted without replication to validate findings. Nurse researchers must be encouraged to build a research program for their career so that the discovery of phenomena in long-term care are useful in application of findings. Perhaps this is one explanation for the lack of applicability of research findings presently—nurses in long-term care realize how shallow published findings are. In addition, explanations for the phenomena studied seem nonrelevant because they do not fit the reality nurses experience in their day to day clinical practice.

FINDINGS FROM A CURRENT SEARCH OF NURSING RESEARCH IN LONG-TERM CARE FACILITIES

To provide an overview of research in gerontological nursing and long-term care facilities completed between the years 1984–1988, Haight reviewed five journals: *Journal of Gerontological Nursing, Geriatric Nursing, Nursing Research, Research in Nursing and Health*, and the *Western Journal of Nursing Research*. While such a review is certainly commendable, it is interesting to this author that so few of the research studies were published in such journals as *Scholarly Inquiry: An International Journal* or *Advances in Nursing Science*. Of the 64 articles identified by Haight, only seven were found in bonafide research journals.

Another concern rises here: Dr. Haight did not identify the criteria by which these five journals were selected for review. Questions that could be raised include: (1) Is the overview as complete as it could be? (2) Why were not journals such as *The Gerontologist* and the *Journal of Gerontology* included in the review since many nurses (including Dr. Haight) have been successful in having their studies published in them? (3) What about review of such journals as *Image, Nursing Times*, and *International Women's Health* for geronotological nursing research? It would have been helpful for this review to have been more inclusive of scholarly publications where sophisticated studies are published under more rigorous scrutiny by non-nurse peer reviewers.

CURRENT TRENDS IN GERONTOLOGICAL NURSING RESEARCH

Identification of the need for more studies on the physical dimension of older residents is highly important and is a strength of the review since, as was noted by Haight, Maslow's hierarchy of needs cannot be met if basic physiological needs are not satisfied to the expectations of the older person. Of particular concern are the feeding and bathing components of care as described so well by Haight. Haight's 15 categories of research that note the advancement of gerontological nursing research efforts toward issues other than studies of attitudes and nurse behaviors reveals a refreshing trend in gerontological nursing research. Unfortunately, too many of the completed studies are limited in size of subjects and generalizability to the nursing arena. This limitation has implications for application of the findings to the clinical settings where nursing care of older adults should benefit from research efforts.

Another factor unearthed by Dr. Haight (in terms of trends on gerontological nursing research) is a lack of preparation in rigorous research skills provided by graduate programs in gerontological nursing. Rather than requiring of the student a rigorously designed research study for graduation from a master's degree program, many of these programs present as optional the completion of a thesis. Consequently, many gerontological nurse graduates who have knowledge and expertise in clinical gerontological nursing fail to understand the research process sufficiently. As a result, they do not possess the competence and confidence to design research studies that could be useful in application of data analysis and findings to promote upgrading of care. This insufficiency becomes critical when coupled with the fact that only 2–3% of master's-prepared nurse graduates continue with advanced education where expertise in research skills is obtained. Nursing educational programs that are eliminating the thesis as a requirement for graduation should reconsider this trend. In light of the data and analysis required to present hard-core cases to legislators for nursing care needs of older adults in various settings—for example, home, hospital, nursing homes, day care centers, extended care facilities, and improvement of holistic care in other institutionalized settings—research skills are a vital and necessary basis.

SUGGESTIONS FOR FUTURE RESEARCH
IN GERONTOLOGICAL NURSING

The most important section of Haight's paper concerns the need for future research. Haight's detailed overview of needs for environment, health promotion and clinical problems, disease prevention, staff and costs, and patient, family, and future nursing practice sets the stage for future research. To illustrate her remarks, Dr. Haight provides discussion regarding the three most important research topics (from her perspective) related to research utilization, end-state

Alzheimer's disease, and nursing home environment. Each of these suggestions makes note of the wide variability of research currently and the tremendous needs for future research to assist in understanding the complexity of care for the older adult.

In this area, specific concerns surround the issue that nursing homes, long-term care (LTC) facilities, remain a vast arena for research but to date have been underutilized for research activities. Perhaps the fault lies with the director of nursing in long-term care not appreciating the value of conducting studies and engaging the nursing staff in the pursuit of knowledge through this medium; or, perhaps the nursing staff have become so routine in their perceptions of the older adult and the provision of care that complacency has set in. As a result, little energy is directed toward new and more effective approaches to upgrading care. Perhaps the problem lies with allocating monies for research activities in the nursing budget when there are so many other pressing and immediate needs. Whatever the reason, it remains clear that more effort must be expended toward improvement of care of older adults in long-term care facilities through research that can be useful in promoting the well being of older adults in these institutions.

OTHER STRENGTHS AND LIMITATIONS
NOTED BY THE RESPONDENT

Strengths

A major strength of Haight's paper included the utilization of the integrated review methodology for the five-year span of research in long-term care as described by Ganong (1984). This approach provides a quick reference to the major findings and research design utilized by researchers. It is this respondent's opinion that, once published, this material will be utilized widely in research circles. Ganong's overview is provided in 25 tables with a format of great practicality. Ganong defines the integrative review method in this way: "An integrative review is defined as one in which the reviewer is primarily interested in inferring generalizations about substantive issues from a set of studies directly bearing on those issues. Such reviews include examination of research support for competing hypothesis, suggestions for new theoretical issues, and identification of needed research" (p.1).

An additional strength of Haight's paper was her suggestions (1) to provide a more comprehensive body of knowledge and (2) to set the research agenda in the 1990s.

Limitations

Limitations of Haight's paper included these elements:

1. The definition of long-term care was too narrow. It did not include the continuity of care concept of home health care as well as nursing home care.

2. Accessibility of nurse researchers into the clinical settings as obstacles to conduction of clinical studies was not addressed. Nurse researchers are not generally welcome in long-term care settings if the Director of Nursing and other nurse personnel are uncomfortable regarding the research process and its applicability to nursing care. The author guides dissertation studies of doctoral students who have repeatedly had difficulties in gaining access to older residents in long-term care facilities, which poses problems in the conducting of rigorously designed studies in such settings. In addition, the problems are compounded when nurses in the facilities are not supportive of the nurse researcher when in the setting and fail to observe the protocols the researcher has in place for conducting the study. These weaknesses were not addressed in Haight's paper but should be noted for presenting an explanation for the limited and fragmented approach to nursing research in long-term care settings.

3. A question raised by this respondent relates to Dr. Haight's interpretative statement. This statement is based on a study of attitudes and knowledge that implied nurse educators would not likely think gerontological nursing education as useful for recruiting nurses into educational programs. Some clarification of this statement would be useful to readers.

CONCLUSION

The paper presented by Dr. Haight is an excellent representation of state-of-the-art gerontological nursing research in long-term care. Use of an integrative review of nursing research methodology presents the material in such a way that a large body of literature is organized for quick reference to design, methodology, and findings. Based on Dr. Haight's presentation, a Delphi study will be conducted by the National League for Nursing Long-Term Care Committee. This study will define the research agenda for the 1990s using the members of the Long-Term Care Committee and the presenters at this invitational conference.

As expert participants in the study, they will determine the research needs to promote the body of knowledge in gerontological nursing and its application for improvement of nursing care to older adults. With this outcome, gerontological nursing will be launched into the next century on a more solid basis for influencing health policy, nursing care, and the improvement of such care to the older adult. With such a thrust, the holistic needs of older adults will be met and the future of gerontological nursing will be more lustrous and influential in all arenas.

REFERENCES

Ganong, L. H. (1984). Integrative review of nursing research. *Research in Nursing and Health*, *10*, 1–11.

4

An Overview of Current Research Relating to Outcomes of Care

Donna Ambler Peters, PhD, RN
Program Officer
The Robert Wood Johnson Foundation
Princeton, NJ

Quality of care is our concern today, and the concern of our society in general. In fact, the issue of quality has become a matter of public debate, the results of which will ultimately shape the delivery of health care. This current wave of concern about quality care focuses not on raising or improving care, but rather on preserving quality while efforts to reduce costs are actualized. The challenge is to provide and monitor quality on behalf of all the diverse groups that demand that quality care exist (i.e., the federal government, providers, and the general public). The key questions are: what is quality and how is it measured?

Defining quality and quality health care is a formidable task. It remains an elusive concept conjuring debates over whether or not it can be defined, or whether it can only be found in the eye of the beholder. However, there is agreement that quality health care does exist if it positively alters the health

The views expressed in this article are solely those of the author and official endorsement by the Robert Wood Johnson Foundation is not intended and should not be inferred.

status of the person receiving it. The purpose of this paper, therefore, is to examine quality in long-term care from the perspective of patient outcomes. This will be accomplished by discussing (1) the measurement of quality in long-term care, (2) the concept of outcome measurement, and (3) examples of current research on outcome measurement in home health care. By first defining the concept of outcome measurement, it is possible to evaluate current research in terms of which parts each study does or does not address.

QUALITY IN LONG-TERM CARE

In order to measure quality in long-term care, three areas are considered: (1) the scope of health care in long-term care; (2) what criteria need to be measured; and (3) a framework for the measurement.

Long-term care covers a wide range of services because of the chronic conditions, disabilities, and dependency state of the elderly population. This vulnerable population is a complex and diverse group. There are several different subgroups such as underserved minorities, the terminally ill, and those recently discharged from the hospital who are recovering from an acute illness. Each subgroup often has different needs and different benefit potentials, thus they may require different services. While it is not the intent of this paper to define long-term care, the elements of health care included in long-term care can be briefly described as: the functional improvement of the client, modifications in the environment that eliminate physical and psychological barriers to the individual's desired autonomy, and issues relating to quality of life.

To try to categorize long-term care under medical diagnosis does not work, and using only technical treatments leaves large care deficits. Nursing is the primary service in long-term care and thus provides the insight necessary to identify the problems of delivering long-term care and the solutions to those problems. It is nursing assessments that yield the most descriptive and valid indicators of the quality of care needed (Lang, 1988).

Other conditions found in the long-term care setting that complicate the delivery of care and the measurement of quality include the use of a large number of unlicensed personnel to give care and the increasing use of high technology. When long-term care is offered at home, even more dilemmas arise. For example, the care provider is a guest in the client's home and only visits on an intermittent basis. It is more difficult here to maintain any type of control over the client's behavior in complying with the prescribed treatment plan. Not only may the client display a specific outcome in spite of the care rendered, but also those contributions to care made by health professionals may be difficult to differentiate from those made by family or the client.

A second area to consider when measuring quality in long-term care is the selection of criteria to be assessed. The criteria chosen to measure quality differs based on the group looking for the assurance of quality: the federal government, health care professionals and organizations, and the client. The federal government's mandate is for quality in the aggregate; its concept of quality focuses on a system to monitor key aspects of care to determine whether or not the care delivered was necessary or appropriate. Measurement of quality could thus consist of utilization criteria such as the number of services and visits delivered and the number of days services were rendered. In contrast, health care professionals and organizations recognize the clinical concept of quality and focus on measuring the delivery of technically correct care. This entails more detailed information that is obtained by developing patient typologies in order to identify patterns of care. Once measures of quality are identified, a mechanism is necessary to assess care provided against those measures and to correct deficiencies.
is necessary to assess care provided against those measures and to correct deficiencies.

The client offers a final perspective on the type of criteria needed to assure quality. Client concerns center on whether or not expected outcomes were achieved and whether or not the client was satisfied with the care received (Lalonde, 1988). Outcomes from this perspective must be client specific and provide feedback to the health care giver for further decision making on providing care. The validity of using patient satisfaction as one of these indicators of quality is a debated issue. It can be argued that patients lack the knowledge to evaluate technical aspects of care or that they may feel intimidated in expressing their opinions because of their dependency on health care givers. Despite arguments, however, several factors have stimulated interest in using patient satisfaction as an assessment of the quality of care. These factors include: (1) consumers are more sophisticated about the type of care they receive; (2) health care providers are becoming more attentive to consumer concerns; and (3) competition for clients has intensified. Furthermore, clients play an important role in defining what constitutes quality care by determining what values should be associated with different outcomes (Cleary & McNeil, 1988).

The third area to consider when measuring quality in long-term care is the framework for the measurement. The most accepted framework for measuring quality is Donabedian's (1987) concept of structure, process, and outcome. Structure addresses the nature of the resources that are assembled to provide health care, process refers to the intermediate products of care (the act of providing care), and outcomes are the end products of care (Berwick & Knapp, 1987).

For the past two decades, most quality assurance work has stressed process of care evaluations and classification of the technical quality of care. The emphasis has now shifted to client outcomes. Academically this is derived from the "health accounting" concepts of the late 1970s; practically it arises from the growing concern about the effects of cost containment on client well-being (Lohr, 1988). The greatest motivation is the federal government's mandate to include clinical outcomes in nursing home and home care surveys. The Omnibus Reconciliation Act (OBRA) of 1987 mandates the development of a resident assessment process, including patient outcome measures, suitable for national use by all nursing home facilities participating in Medicare and Medicaid. Assessment findings will be used as the basis for planning and evaluating the care that is provided to all patients and by 1993 will also serve as the core of the survey process used to monitor care provided in nursing home facilities. OBRA 1987 also charges the Secretary of Health and Human Services to develop an instrument to be used by home health agency surveyors that will assess the extent to which the quality of the scope of services furnished by an agency attained the highest practical functional capacity for its clients. The new process will use outcome measures of medical, nursing, and rehabilitation care.

Although the current focus of quality is on outcome measurement, it must be remembered that the elements of structure, process, and outcome have meaning only in the context of the others and taken alone are not a valid indicator of quality. Instead, each are components in a chain, bound to one another by causal connections (Wyszewianski, 1988). Outcomes, for example, do not tell precisely what may have gone wrong and who was responsible. In fact, a client may display a specific outcome despite the health care received or the lack thereof. Outcomes by nature are delayed, less sensitive, and less specific. However, outcomes have the advantage of being comprehensible and reflective. They reflect all antecedent care including clinical judgment and skill as well as the contribution of clients to their own care (Donabedian, 1987).

The complexities of measuring quality in long-term care cannot be overstated. It has already been mentioned that long-term care deals with a diverse population and is not defined by the medical model. In addition, long-term care: (1) offers various goals; (2) is provided in diversely structured settings; (3) frequently is delivered in fragmentation; and (4) does not lend itself to highly measurable criteria. Thus, making adaptations in quality measurement from acute care is inappropriate, and developing valid, meaningful outcomes becomes a challenge.

CONCEPTS OF OUTCOME MEASUREMENT

As a construct, patient outcomes are immensely complex. Three components to be considered are: (1) reliability and validity, (2) characteristics, and (3) elements of measurement (Lohr, 1988).

Reliability and validity determine whether the given outcome measures produce the same results when the same cases are assessed more than once and whether they actually measure what they purport to measure.

The four characteristics of client outcomes include: (1) dimension of health, (2) definiteness, (3) timing, and (4) correlation of outcome to processes of care (Lohr, 1988). Dimension of health refers to the aspect of health being considered. If the scope of health care includes physical, emotional, environmental, and quality of life issues, however defined, then outcomes would need to be developed for each of these aspects in order to measure all the dimensions. Definiteness of outcomes refers to the level of objectivity or subjectivity of the outcome. Hospital readmission rates, for example, are an objective outcome. However, as long-term care quality indicator, they are ambiguous because hospitalization may not always be an undesired outcome if a client can benefit from monitoring or treatment in an acute-care setting. Subjective outcomes include symptomatology such as pain.

Another inherent characteristic of outcome measures is that they denote changes in status from one point in time to another. Client status at one point in time is not an outcome measure in itself. If the first measurement of client status occurs on admission to long-term care, a decision must be made about the intervals for taking other measurements. For example, is the outcome measurement made at time of discharge or several weeks later when the client/family have been on their own and the effects of learning/nonlearning may be more evident. In actuality, the most effective way to review quality would be to track clients through an episode of illness rather than to concentrate attention on just one setting. However, the responsibility for assuring quality care rests with the organization providing that care. Therefore, interim outcomes should at least be measured as a client moves from one setting to another.

The final characteristic of outcome measures is the directness of the relationship of outcome to processes of care. The relationship between process and outcome indicators is vague. There are some outcome indicators, however, such as fulfilled unmet needs, compliance with medications, and improved client knowledge that can be more closely related to the processes of care than other long-term results such as restoration of a particular health or functional state. The longer the period of observation required, the more tenuous the connection between outcomes and processes of care.

The third component to the construct of patient outcomes concerns the types of elements to be considered in measurement. These types include (1) purpose of measurment, (2) the agent responsible for analysis and interpretation, (3) source of information, and (4) mode of data collection. (Lohr, 1988).

Purpose of Measurement

The three main purposes for measuring outcomes are related to the group (i.e., federal government, health care professionals and organizations, or the client) interested in the quality measurement. These purposes are: (1) to establish a screening system to identify potential substandard services; (2) to isolate patterns of care across many similar patients that could determine the impact of cost containment measures; and (3) to evaluate care for an individual patient as feedback for further decision making. It should be noted that in order to isolate patterns of care across patients, a patient typology is required to aggregate groups of homogeneous patients.

Agent Responsible for Analysis and Interpretation

The agent responsible for analysis and interpretation of outcomes will most likely be the group interested in the quality measurement—the client, the provider organization, or a regulator such as the federal government. The client will be interested in how well his or her expected outcomes were achieved. The people and organizations that provide the care actually establish the quality and also view it in a personal, individualized manner. Regulatory agencies, on the other hand, tend to look at quality in the aggregate. They are interested in crude measures of quality in order to establish a system of checks and balances to identify and stop substandard or abusive services, monitor utilization, or define policy and economic issues.

Source of Information

This is especially important in long-term care because documented data elements are incomplete and because long-term care is still evolving. Possible sources include the client, proxies for the client (such as the caregiver), charts, and insurance claims records. The focus in acute care has been on nonintrusive outcome measures (such as mortality) that can be gathered from insurance claims records. However, in long-term care, death may be the desired outcome; therefore, care must be taken when using this type of outcome.

Mode of Data Collection

Closely related to source of information, mode of data collection is important because of the lack of detailed data bases on the condition of and the care provided to clients. Data are neither uniform nor easily accessed. Abstraction and errors in recording are long recognized problems (Davis, 1987). Choices for data collection include client interview, questionnaire, and chart review.

Finally, in considering client outcomes, the factor of justified variations or exceptions must also be taken into account. These exceptions must be considered for each outcome to determine if failure to achieve a health outcome represents inappropriate care. Examples of exceptions include a client's refusal of services, a client's move to a different service area, or a client's intractable pain.

EXAMPLES OF CURRENT RESEARCH RELATING TO OUTCOME MEASUREMENT

As much as quality outcome measurement is in the forefront today, little has been done to develop outcomes in long-term care. The National Center for Health Services Research has had a call out for proposals in home health care, including the developing and testing of methods for measuring patient outcomes. As of December 1988, few proposals have been received and none have been funded. There are several individual agencies attempting to incorporate client outcomes into their care process and developing tools to evaluate their success. However, these individual attempts are generally not validated using the research process and they will not be addressed here. The studies presented are not exhaustive, but rather most representative of the work being done, especially in the area of home health care.

One of the earlier studies looking at client-specific criteria is the system of patient problem classification developed by the Visiting Nurse Association of Omaha (Simmons, 1980). The original design was developed with funding from the Division of Nursing of the Department of Health and Human Services (DHHS). The system delineates a nursing diagnosis taxonomy for patients receiving community health care. The diagnoses are divided into the four domains (environmental, psychosocial, psychological, and health behaviors) that are of importance to community health nurses. Client data bases (n = 125) from agencies in four geographic areas were used to validate the occurrence of these health problems and the supporting signs and symptoms. An example of a problem label is: Circulation: Impairment, which would be used for a client exhibiting edema, cramping, decreased pulses, cyanosis, a temperature change in the affected area, varicosities, syncopal episodes, abnormal blood pressure readings, a pulse deficit, an irregular heart rate, an excessively rapid/slow heart rate, anginal pain, or abnormal heart sounds (see Figure 1) (Simmons, 1980).

Expected outcomes and criterion measures were developed and field tested for each of the problem labels, although they were never widely disseminated. In New Jersey, these outcomes were revised and published by the New Jersey Home Health Agency Assembly, Inc. (Cell et al., 1987). Figure 1 also shows the outcomes established for the client problem of circulation.

More recently, under a third contract with the Division of Nursing, the Visiting Nurse Association of Omaha (Simmons, 1986) revised the original taxonomy (the system now delineates 44 client problems), developed an intervention scheme, and developed a problem rating scale for outcomes. Outcomes are rated for each problem on a five-point Likert scale using the concepts of knowledge, behavior, and status. Each concept is operationalized for a client problem using the signs and symptoms associated with the problem. The appropriate outcome for each concept is selected for an individual patient. This rating scale was field tested in four sites. Interrater reliability ranged from a low of 41 to a high of 65 for exact matches and from a low of 83 to a high of 96 for matches with a difference of 1. Results of the field test were used to make final modifications in the scheme (Martin, 1988).

An example of this scale can be demonstrated using a client with the symptom of edema. A rating would be made for the concept of knowledge, behavior, and status. A client rated as a 3 under knowledge, or having average knowledge, would be aware that elevation of feet increases comfort level. For behavior, a rating of 1, or having inappropriate behavior, would be defined as the client unwilling to put on TED hose. Finally, having no pedal edema and slight ankle edema would result in a rating of 4, minimal signs/symptoms, on the status scale (Simmons, 1986). Thus, two clients with edema could have dissimilar outcomes, that is, another client could have a rating of 5 for knowledge (client explains that good circulation results in no edema), 4 for behavior (client wears TED hose when legs are swollen), and 2 for status (nonpitting edema to feet, pitting edema to ankles), respectively (Simmons, 1986). Although this system is useful for purposes of evaluating the care of individual clients, it does not readily allow for the evaluation of patterns of care across the grouping of clients.

In contrast is the work done by Dr. Bernadette Lalonde in conjunction with the Home Care Association of Washington and funded by the Health Care

Figure 1
Client Outcomes for Circulation: Impairment

NAME_____ DATE: _____

PHYSIOLOGICAL

24. CIRCULATION: Impairment
    - 01. edema
    - 02. cramping/pain of extremities
    - 03. decreased pulses
    - 04. discoloration of skin/cyanosis
    - 05. temperature change in affected area
    - 06. varicosities
    - 07. syncopal episodes
    - 08. abnormal blood pressure reading
    - 09. pulse deficit
    - 10. irregular heart rate
    - 11. excessively rapid/slow heart rate
    - 12. reports anginal pain
    - 13. abnormal heart sounds
    - 14. other

Client Outcome: PREVENTION   MAINTENANCE   IMPROVEMENT

	Time Frame	Evaluation Date and Summary

a. Accurate and Timely Prevention/
   Treatment Regime

   V = _____
   D = _____
   W = _____

   1. does exercises
   2. demonstrates a balance between rest activity
   3. elevates legs
   4. utilizes safety measures
   5. does skin care
   6. uses support stockings/wrappings
   7. follows diet
   8. takes medications per schedule
   9. other

b. Changed/Stable Circulatory Status

   V = _____
   D = _____
   W = _____

   1. reports less palpitations
   2. heart rate is more regular
   3. reports decreased headaches
   4. reports decreased or no dizziness
   5. reports less/no pain
   6. has less/no edema
   7. shows improved skin appearance/temperature
   8. has improved pedal/tibial pulses
   9. TPR is reduced
   10. BP is reduced
   11. weight is decreased/increased
   12. other

c. Express interest/understanding of current/
   potential circulatory status

   V = _____
   D = _____
   W = _____

   1. expresses desire to prevent/decrease circulatory impairment
   2. verbalizes risk factors
   3. verbalizes causes of circulation impairment
   4. verbalizes treatment options
   5. states impact of treatment versus nontreatment
   6. other

d. Other

   V = _____
   D = _____
   W = _____   Signed _____

Source: *Components for the successful use of the Omaha classification system:* Home Health Agency Assembly of New Jersey, Inc., New Jersey: 1987.

Finance Administration (HCFA) (Lalonde, 1988). The intent of this project was to develop seven broad-based client-centered outcome scales applicable to *all* home health care clients regardless of diagnosis or nursing problem. The scales are: (1) Taking Prescribed Medications as Prescribed; (2) General Symptom Distress; (3) Discharge Status; (4) Caregiver Strain; (5) Functional Status; (6) Knowledge of Major Health Problem/Diagnosis; and (7) Physiological Indicator Scale. Each scale is constructed differently, and (with the exception of the Discharge Status Scale) is meant to be applied by interview within three visits prior to the client's discharge from service. Clients are not differentiated, therefore, data is aggregated on all home care clients even though this is a diverse population. Interrater reliability and face, content, and construct validity were established for each scale. Over a six-week period, each scale was tested on approximately 120–190 randomly selected clients in 5–7 home care agencies across Washington State representative of the broad home care agency spectrum (VNA, proprietary, large, small). Explicit implementation and scoring instructions were developed to ensure that all home care agencies would implement and score the scales in the same way.

One example of these scales is the General Symptom Distress Scale (GSDS) (Lalonde, 1987) (see Figure 2). The GSDS covers general symptoms considered important for home care and which should be monitored and managed for all clients. In addition, these are symptoms which either occur frequently in the home care population or are very distressing to the client and can be easily managed. They are: pain, nausea/vomiting, bowel problems (e.g., diarrhea, constipation, incontinence), urinary/bladder problems (e.g., retention, incontinence), cough, respiratory difficulties (e.g., shortness of breath, congestion), swelling/fluid retention, skin problems (e.g., rashes, sores, open wounds), speech problems (e.g., swallowing, making yourself understood), mood (e.g., anxiety, depression), and activity level (e.g., weakness, coordination, endurance). Each symptom is rated on a five-point scale, 0 = no problem and 4 = symptom is present and remains distressing for more than half the time of wakefulness. The scale takes only 10 minutes to complete. It is recommended that every agency patient be rated on admission, midway through service, and at discharge. The result is both individual data (i.e., how well a client is progressing and which clients need attention) and aggregate data. The aggregate data informs the agency administration how well the agency is managing symptoms across clients (i.e., the number and percent of clients with scores of 3 or 4 for each symptom).

The remaining studies utilize a classification system to stratify clients into groups that are homogeneous with respect to quality indicators that apply.

The first system, the Rehabilitation Potential Patient Classification System, was developed by Daubert (1979), and classifies patients into one of five patient groups according to each patient's rehabilitation potential regardless of diagnosis or problems.

Daubert's system represents an early attempt to measure quality of home care services. Although it is mostly a process audit, it does group clients according to their outcome objective. The five categories of outcome objectives are recovery, self-care, rehabilitation, maintenance, and terminal. The categories are defined by specific criteria including an overall outcome objective and a number of suboutcome objectives. For example, an overall objective for the recovery category as adapted by the VNA of Eastern Montgomery County is: Client will achieve complete recovery from illness, or client's immediate health need, which prompted admission to service, will be eliminated. Subobjectives for the category include: (1) client/family will demonstrate ability to assume responsibility for ongoing medical supervision and (2) client/family will demonstrate an understanding of prescribed diet (Harris, Peters, & Yuan, 1987). The original use of the system was to measure the client against all outcome criteria simultaneously. However, at least one agency has now begun using each subobjective as an additional outcome measurement. Data on the success of this use is not yet available.

Other studies represent works in progress with no final product available as yet. For example, there is a study being done at the University of Colorado Health Sciences Center by Dr. Peter Shaughnessy et al. and funded by the Robert Wood Johnson Foundation. The purpose of this study is to develop a set of quality indicators, primarily outcome indicators, that could potentially be used to monitor/assure quality in home health care. This set of outcomes will be designed to include a representative spectrum of outcomes for the home care population.

Based on potential home health clients, a taxonomy for home health care is being developed using patient age categories and needs for care in the home setting. The needs are: acute/subacute, chronic, and preventive. For each need category, clients are categorized by age—either elderly, nonelderly adult, maternal/newborn, and pediatric. For each client group (e.g., elderly, chronic) a set of quality outcome indicators that would apply to all the clients in the group is being developed. The three major groupings of outcomes being used are utilization measures, client status outcomes, and client satisfaction status. The outcomes are being established using staff expertise and an expert panel in this preliminary effort to develop quality outcome indicators in home care. Shaughnessy has also been funded by HCFA to develop outcome-based quality measures for the Medicare population receiving home care services. Although this project has been funded, work has not yet begun.

Additional work in this field was begun by this paper's author. Peters' (1989)

Figure 2
General Symptom Distress Scale

Client's Chart Number _____

Length of Stay Last Admission _____ Days

Primary Diagnosis _____

CIRCLE THE SYMPTOMS THE CLIENT SAYS HE/SHE HAS EXPERIENCED WITHIN THE PAST MONTH

SYMPTOMS

Pain	Nausea/ Vomiting	Bowel Problems (diarrhea, constipation, incontinence)	Urinary/ Bladder Problems (retention, incontinence)	Cough	Respiratory Difficulties (shortness of breath, congestion)

Swelling/Fluid Retention	Skin Problems (raw areas, rashes, sores, open wounds, itching)	Speech Problems (difficulty speaking, swallowing, making yourself understood)	Mood (anxiety, depression)	Activity Level (weakness, lack of coordination, lack of endurance)

(WRITE IN CIRCLED SYMPTOMS) ▲ ▲ FOR EACH SYMPTOM ASK	Col 1	Col 2	Col 3	Col 4	Col 5	Col 6	Col 7	Col 8
"Are you currently taking a medication for your (name of symptom) or taking any actions for it?"								

"In the past 3 days, has your (name of symptom) been a problem for you?"

(IF YES)   (IF NO ▲ ► STOP FINAL
▶   SCORE = 1. GO TO NEXT
                SYMPTOM)

"Can your (name of symptom) be easily ignored?"

(IF NO)   (IF YES ▲ ► STOP. FINAL
▶   SCORE = 2. GO TO NEXT
                SYMPTOM)

"In a 24-hour period, does your (name of symptom) bother you less ☐ than one-half of the time you are awake or more ☐ than one-half of the time you are awake?" (Check the appropriate box. If exactly one-half of the time, consider as more than one-half of the time.)

(IF LESS THAN ONE-HALF OF THE TIME, FINAL SCORE = 3. IF ONE-HALF THE TIME OR MORE THAN ONE-HALF THE TIME, FINAL SCORE = 4. GO TO NEXT SYMPTOM)

FINAL SCORE EACH COLUMN _____

Number of circled symptoms _____   Time to complete scale _____ minutes

Note: Verbatim instructions to the interviewer have been deleted. See text for description of instructions. The *General Symptom Distress Scale* is used to measure the distress caused by 11 general symptoms experienced by home care clients.

Source: *Quality Review Bulletin* (1987) Vol. 13, p. 244. Copyright 1989 by the Joint Commission on Accreditation of Healthcare Organizations, Chicago. Reprinted with permission.

Figure 3
Community Health Intensity Rating Scale
Parameter Definitions

ENVIRONMENTAL DOMAIN

Finances

Available financial resources, including employment status, of an individual/family reflecting the adequacy/availability of income related to financial obligations.

Housing: Safety, Health

Condition of patient's home/neighborhood including availability of necessary facilities and transportation to those facilities.

PSYCHOSOCIAL DOMAIN

Community Networking

Individual's/family's knowledge and use of community resources/services.

Family system

Interpersonal relationships within the household (primary unit) and/or with relatives, friends, and significant others outside the household such as church members, social group members, and fellow employees.

Emotional Response

Expression of feelings including sexual concerns, grief, spiritual beliefs, depression, anxiety, and behavioral outcomes that arise from an individual's/family's perception of self as it relates to a change in health.

Individual Growth and Development

Early/adult life development of cognitive, physical, and social tasks including ability to speak, read, and write.

PHYSIOLOGICAL DOMAIN

Sensory Function

The body function concerned with the use of senses to include vision, hearing, taste, touch, smell, proprioception, and an individual's perception of pain.

Respiratory/ Circulatory Function	The body functions concerned with (1) the transfer of gases to meet ventilatory needs and (2) the supply of blood to body tissues via the cardiovascular system.
Neuromusculo- skeletal Function	The body functions concerned with integration and direction of body regulatory processes related to gross and fine motor movements including level of consciousness, mental status, speech patterns, muscle strength, coordination, skeletal integrity, and degree of physical independence/mobility.
Reproductive Function	The body function concerned with menstruation, family planning, fertility, pregnancy, lactation, and impediments of sexual activity. Included are sexual organs and secondary sexual characteristics such as breasts.
Digestive/ Elimination	The ability to ingest food and fluids, utilize nutrients and excrete waste products from the body.
Structural Integrity	The character and intactness of the body's protective mechanisms including skin and/or the immunological system.

HEALTH BEHAVIORS DOMAIN

Nutrition	An individual's/family's selection, preparation, and consumption of nutrients including cultural and health factors.
Personal Habits	An individual's/family's management of personal health related activities. It includes sleep–activity patterns, personal hygiene, and avoidance of harmful materials. It addresses patient/family habits or preferences, not ability to do ADLs.
Health Management	An individual's/family's management of their own health status including their perception of health and their motivation to strive for an optimal level of wellness.

Source: Originally published in Peters, D.A. (1988). *Examples of existing quality assurance programs in home health care: A hospital-based agency.* In C. Meisenheimer (Ed.), *Quality assurance in home care* (p. 255). Rockville, MD: Aspen.

Reprinted from *Quality Assurance for Home Health Care* by C.G. Meisenheimer, p. 255, with permission of Aspen Publishers, Inc., © 1989.

work incorporates the work of the Visiting Nurse Association of Omaha. Instead of 44 client problems, the scope of home health care is defined using 15 Community Health Parameters categorized within the four domains of the Omaha Classification System (environmental, psychosocial, physiological, and health behaviors). These parameters are: (1) Environmental Domain: finances, housing, safety, health; (2) Psychosocial Domain: community networking, family system, emotional response, individual growth and development; (3) Physiological Domain: sensory function, respiratory and circulatory function, neuromusculoskeletal function, reproductive function, digestive/elimination, structural integrity; and (4) Health Behaviors Domain: nutrition, personal habits, and health management. (See Figure 3 for Parameter Definitions.)

Use of these parameters provides a mechanism of organizing data in home health care using a nursing model which is congruent with the services that are being rendered. In essence, the combined content of the 15 community health parameters describes home health care within the definition of long-term care in the community. In addition, these parameters have been incorporated within a conceptual framework for community health practice (see Figure 4). The 15 parameters are identified as the Community Health Nursing Intensity Construct. The rationale for using a conceptual framework is fourfold:

- It is useful for organizing all the components of an agency—clinical practice, administration, and the quality assurance program.
- It defines and articulates the practice of nursing and thus supports nurses in their daily practice.
- It provides a common data base which facilitates communication within an agency and prevents confusion over terminology.
- It provides a structure for quality assurance that not only defines terms but also visualizes the relationship of structure, process, and outcome, and provides the organization for doing something about the results obtained after care is measured against standards.

Once the conceptual framework was developed, it became obvious that clinical quality indicators for care did not exist. Thus, preliminary process and outcome indicators are being developed to cover the generic content areas within each parameter. For example, one of the content areas in the nutrition parameter is intake. A process indicator for this area would read: Patients with impairment in intake will have: (a) monitoring of intake and potential barriers to intake and (b) provision of supplemental intake. The outcome measurement would be: The client will demonstrate sufficient intake and/or potential barriers to intake will be minimized or eliminated. These indicators are preliminary and have not yet been field tested.

Figure 4

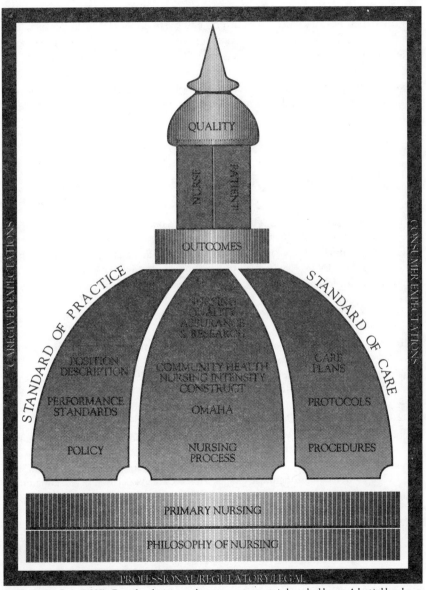

Source: Peters, D.A. (1988). *Examples of existing quality assurance programs in home health care: A hospital based agency*. In C. Meisenheimer (Ed.), *Quality assurance in home care*. Rockville, Md. Aspen, pg. 253.
Adapted from Journal of Nursing Quality Assurance, Vol. 2, No. 1., p.31, with permission of Aspen Publishers, Inc. © November 1987

CONCLUSION

This paper has discussed the current emphasis on outcome indicators, the complexities of the outcome construct, and some of the studies that have been or are being conducted. It is obvious that although the need for outcomes for various categories of clients in long-term care is present, the development of them is slow and complicated. Researchers, however, are challenged to continue to develop and test valid outcome measures for this population; the federal mandate is already in place.

REFERENCES

Berwick, D.M., & Knapp, M.G. (1987). Theory and practice for measuring health care quality. *Health Care Financing Review*, annual supple., 49–55.

Cell, P., et al. (1987). *Components for the successful use of the Omaha Classification System*. New Jersey: Home Health Agency Assembly of New Jersey, Inc.

Cleary, P.D., & McNeil, B.J. (1988). Patient satisfaction as an indicator of quality care. *Inquiry*, *25*(1), 25–36.

Daubert, E.A. (1979). Patient classification system and outcome criteria. *Nursing Outlook*, *27*, 450–454.

Davis, F.A. (1987). Quality of health care measurement: A research priority. *Health Care Financing Review*, annual supple., 1–3.

Donabedian, A. (1987). Commentary on some studies of the quality of care. *Health Care Financing Review*, annual supple., 75–85.

Harris, M.D., Peters, D.A., & Yuan, J. (1987). Relating quality and cost in a home health care agency. *Quarterly Review Bulletin*, *13*, 175–181.

Lalonde, B. (1987). The General symptom distress scale: A home care outcome measure. *Quarterly Review Bulletin*, *13*, 243–250.

Lalonde, B. (1988). *Quality assurance manual of The Home Care Association of Washington* (2nd edition). Washington, DC: The Home Care Association of Washington.

Lalonde, B. (1988). Assuming the quality of home care via the assessment of client outcomes. *Caring*, *7*(1), 20–24.

Lang, N. (1988). Non-hospital, non-physician review. *The Ampra Review*, *5*(4), 1–2.

Lohr, K.N. (1988). Outcome measurement: Concepts and questions. *Inquiry*, *25*(1), 37–50.

Martin, K. (1988). Personal communication.

Peters, D.A. (1989). Examples of existing quality assurance programs in home health care. In C.G. Meisenheimer (Ed.), *Quality assurance for home health care*. Rockville, MD: Aspen.

Simmons, D.A. (1980). A classification scheme for client problems in community health nursing. (DHHS Publication No. HRA 80-16). Washington, DC: United States Government Printing Office.

Simmons, D.A. (1986). *Client management information system for community health nursing agencies.* (NTS Assession No. HRP-0907023). Springfield, VA: National Technical Information Service.

Wyszewianski, L. (1988). Quality of care: Past achievements and future challenges. *Inquiry, 25*(1), 13–22.

5

Response to: "Current Research Relating to Outcomes of Care"

Marjorie K. Bauman, MS, RN
Research Associate
Center for Health Policy Research
and
Center for Health Services Research
University of Colorado Health Sciences Center
Denver, CO

I want to take this opportunity to thank the National League for Nursing and Ross Laboratories for their interest in quality measurement in long-term care and for inviting me to participate in this conference. It is my pleasure to comment on Dr. Donna Peters' paper on quality outcome measurement in long-term care. Dr. Peters' interest and personal efforts in the areas of quality assurance and measurement are to be commended.

Dr. Peters provided an excellent overview of current efforts in outcome measurement in long-term care, particularly home health care. My remarks will also focus on home health services, but many points have potential application to the nursing home industry as well.

I would like to emphasize three major points in outcome measurement in the home health care field:

1. The unique nature of home health care.

2. The complexities in quality measurement of home health services.

3. The proper balance of structure, process, and outcome measures.

THE UNIQUE NATURE OF HOME HEALTH CARE

Home health care is unique because patients represent a broad spectrum of patient types, from the unstable, post-acute patient who may need high-tech services in the home to the chronic care patient who needs more personal care and support services with only occasional clinical assessment by a licensed provider.

The home setting—the patient's own residence—also sets it apart from other types of care. Because patients are dispersed, it is difficult to observe them to monitor the quality of care provided. In addition, because care is given in the patient's home, the health care provider visits in the therapeutic environment only briefly, thereby decreasing the control the provider might exercise over the patient's behavior. The clinician may provide high-quality teaching to the patient, but he or she is not present to reinforce learning or facilitate improved retention and increased knowledge, all of which potentially affect patient adherence to the treatment plan and, therefore, any measurable change in patient behavior. Thus, the provider has the added responsibility of teaching the treatment regimen to families.

Because a great deal of patient care is given by families or others in the home, an effective patient support system is critically important in home care. Stresses and strains in this support system, perhaps created by the patient's disease or disability, affect the coping abilities of both patient and family/caregiver and, ultimately, patient progress and outcomes.

COMPLEXITIES IN QUALITY MEASUREMENT

The second major issue is the complexity of measuring quality of care provided in the home. As Dr. Peters pointed out, the patient population is difficult to categorize; patients and their conditions are quite diverse (e.g., post-acute, rehabilitative, chronic, terminal). Because of this diversity, patient problems are not adequately described by any particular model (e.g., medical diagnosis, nursing care problem).

In addition, a variety of goals are emphasized by a variety of interested parties. For example, the patient may want personable and unhurried care providers who are willing to "go the extra mile," the provider agency may want clinicians to demonstrate proficiency in technical skills, and the third-party payer may be interested in the cost-effectiveness of quality care. In order to adequately deal with this complexity, one must link quality indicators to patient conditions through the use of a patient classification system in which patient groups are relatively homogeneous from the perspective of quality indicators that apply to each group.

STRUCTURE, PROCESS, AND OUTCOME MEASURES

The third major issue in developing quality measures is the need to properly balance structure, process, and outcome measures in long-term care quality assurance in general, and, specifically, in home health care. As Dr. Peters pointed out, each approach (i.e., structure, process, outcome) taken alone is not a valid indicator of quality. Rather, each is a component of a chain of causal connections.

Structure Measures

When used in conjunction with outcome and process measures, structure indicators may play an important role in quality assurance for long-term care. Structure standards establish the presence of organizational elements thought to be necessary to provision of acceptable care (e.g., staff qualifications or training). Compliance with structure standards, however, does not assure that organizational capability is translated into good patient care. It may even be argued that compliance on paper with structure measures may indeed detract from the provision of patient care because of the administrative burden imposed by such standards.

Process Measures

Process measures have the appeal of applying directly to services administered by a specific provider. They help elucidate aspects of care that are deficient (e.g., initial patient assessment), and they more readily translate into recommendations for improvement (e.g., standards for adequate initial assessment of patient, support systems, and home environment). Process measures also may supplement outcome measures by making it possible to attribute particular outcomes (good or bad) to patient care administered by a particular provider. Process measures (i.e., measures of the quality of care provided) may even be preferable to outcome measures (i.e., measures of change in health status over time) for evaluating the quality of care among patients for whom outcomes are difficult to define (e.g., mentally impaired patients) or difficult to measure (e.g., the terminally ill). Determining process standards, however, can be difficult when system-wide constraints exist that render optimal standards unattainable (e.g., limitations on availability of qualified staff).

Outcome Measures

The conceptual appeal of outcome measures for evaluating quality is rooted in the premise that health care is intended to affect an individual's health status. Since home health care affects many different facets of an individual's health, outcome indicators can relate to several domains of health as well (e.g., physiological status, functional status, satisfaction, health-related knowledge). Outcome measures tend to reflect the impact of the total patient care environment, thus assessing the quality of care across multiple providers rather than the care provided by one individual or agency.

In focusing on outcomes of care, one must take into consideration that factors other than the care provided might contribute to outcome. This is especially true in home health care where the provider agency has relatively little control over the total care environment of the patient. In some instances, home health clinicians may have great difficulty influencing patient outcomes. Selecting a blend of global measures that apply to all patients (e.g., unplanned physician office visit) and focused measures that have a direct relationship to care delivered to specific types of patients (e.g., wound healing in the postsurgical patient) can alleviate some problems. Risk factors (e.g., patient living alone) can then be taken into consideration through patient stratification and, if necessary, case mix adjustment.

OTHER RESEARCH

The Policy Center and Center for Health Services Research at the University of Colorado conduct research and analysis as well as provide technical assistance on topics such as quality assurance, cost containment, reimbursement, and regulation. The most significant focus of our research is in the long-term care field, both nursing home and home health care. The Center for Health Services Research is conducting numerous studies in long-term care, including the project that Dr. Peters mentioned, on monitoring the quality of home health care, funded by the Robert Wood Johnson Foundation. The study team for this six-month project, entitled "A Study to Identify Indicators for Home Health Care," is now concluding its conceptual work.

The Robert Wood Johnson Foundation project consisted of conceptual work on quality indicator development, primarily outcome indicators of quality home health care. In this project, we had a very broad focus of patient age (i.e., infant to elder) and patient condition (e.g., post-acute recovery, rehabilitation, maintenance, chronic conditions, and primary prevention needs). The key to success of this conceptual project was multidisciplinary clinical input from experts in home health care and public health. Together we determined various types of quality indicators, including: a mix of utilization outcomes; health status outcomes, not only of physical and functional status, but also of psychosocial status; patient satisfaction; and patient/family knowledge.

The Center for Health Policy Research also is conducting two other related studies. The center is in its second year of a four-year study, entitled "A Study of Home Health Care Quality and Cost Under Capitated and Fee-For-Service Payment Systems," funded by the Health Care Financing Administration (HCFA). This is a national empirical evaluation of service utilization, quality, and cost of Medicare home health care under capitated (i.e., health maintenance organizations and competitive medical plans) and noncapitated (i.e., fee-for-service) payment systems.

The policy center's second major study in home health care is "Development of Outcome-Based Quality Measures for Home Health Services," also funded by HCFA. This project, in its first of four years, is being conducted to develop, validate, and empirically refine measures of quality of home health care. These measures will be of practical value to the Medicare program in assuring the quality of Medicare-paid home health services.

CONCLUSION

Quality assurance in home health care is in its infancy. Individuals in both research and service sectors are wrestling with the very issues presented here.

Dr. Peters' own research efforts in quality measurement of outcomes of care as well as those mentioned in these presentations are examples of projects aimed at validly and reliably measuring the impact of home health care services on the patient.

RELATED LITERATURE

Bauman, M.K., Kramer, A.M., Shaughnessy, P.W., & Schlenker, R.E. (1988). *Literature and program review of quality assurance systems related to home health care.* Denver, CO: Center for Health Policy Research.

Donabedian, A. (1980). *The definition of quality and approaches to its assessment.* Ann Arbor, MI: Health Administration Press.

Institute of Medicine, Committee on Nursing Home Regulation. (1986). *Improving quality of care in nursing homes.* Washington, DC: National Academy Press.

Kramer, A.M., Shaughnessy, P.W., Bauman, M.K., & Winston, C.L. (1988). *Quality measurement and patient classification for home health care.* Denver, CO: Center for Health Policy Research.

Lalonde, B. (1988). Assuring the quality of home care via the assessment of client outcomes. *Caring, 7*(1), 20–24.

Martin, K., & Scheet, N. (1988). The Omaha system: Providing a framework for assuring quality of home care. *Home Healthcare Nurse, 6*(3), 24–28.

Peters, D. (1988). Quality care: Quality documentation. *Caring, 7*(10), 30–35.

Rinke, L.T. (Ed.). (1987). *Outcome measures in home care, volume 1, research.* New York: National League for Nursing.

Shaughnessy, P.W., & Kurowski, B. (1982). Quality assurance through reimbursement. *Health Services Research, 17*(2), 157–183.

Shaughnessy, P.W. (1985). Long-term care research and public policy. *Health Services Research, 20*(4), 489–499.

6

The Environment and Quality of Care in Long-Term Care Institutions

Jeanie Kayser-Jones, PhD, RN, FAAN*
Professor
Department of Physiological Nursing,
School of Nursing
Medical Anthropology Program, School of Medicine
University of California
San Francisco, CA

The study of environment and behavior has captured the attention of research scientists from many disciplines. In recent years, understanding the effects of the environment on the elderly and searching for optimal environments for the elderly has been a major concern in social gerontology (Kahana, 1982). Despite the availability of research findings, however, there has been limited application of these findings to the care of the institutionalized elderly.

---
*This research was supported in part by a grant from the National Institute on Aging (NIH), grant No. AG05073.

ENVIRONMENT AND AGING: THEORETICAL FRAMEWORK

The environment has been defined as "surroundings—especially those affecting people's lives" (Oxford American Dictionary, 1980). This broad definition includes all our surroundings (e.g., the air we breathe, the freeways we drive on, social relationships, the climate, and disease-carrying organisms). Some investigators have tried to distinguish between the man-made environment, the natural environment, the social environment, and the symbolic environment. They have been forced to acknowledge, however, that the environment is none of these things independently, but rather that it is a result of the constant interaction between the natural and man-made components of the environment, social processes, relationships, and interactions between individuals and groups (Lindheim & Syme, 1983).

Several models have been developed in an attempt to understand and predict the effects of the environment on older people and some investigators have attempted to define optimal environments (Kahana, 1974; Lawton, 1975; Lawton & Nahemow, 1973; Moos, 1980; Moos & Lemke, 1985). While investigators agree that the environment has an important effect on the well being and quality of life for the elderly, systematic guidelines for providing an optimal environment to meet the needs of the elderly have largely been absent, and conceptual approaches for understanding how the environment affects older people have been limited (Kahana, 1982).

Most studies have focused on four major features of the environment: physical characteristics, the organizational climate, the personal and suprapersonal environment, and the social–psychological milieu.

The physical characteristics of an environment include, for example, the architectural design, color, lighting, and space. The organizational aspects include items such as policy, staffing, and financing, as well as the presence or absence of mechanisms such as a resident's council for residents to participate in the planning of their care and airing of grievances.

Lawton (1982) defines the personal environment by way of significant others, who constitute the major one-to-one social relationships of an individual (e.g., family members, friends and work associates), and the suprapersonal environment by way of modal characteristics of all the people in physical proximity to an individual (e.g., the predominant race or the mean age of other residents in a person's neighborhood).

The social–psychological milieu refers to the norms, values, activities, philosophy of the administration, attitudes and beliefs of the caregivers, and the personal interactions of all who are a part of the institution (e.g., residents, staff, and visitors).

Conceptual Framework: Moos

For the purpose of this paper, I will briefly present a conceptual framework developed by Moos (1980) for examining specialized residential settings and how they influence older people. In this model (see Figure 1), the environmental system and the personal system interact to produce cognitive appraisal and activation or motivation. These mediating variables influence one's efforts to adapt or cope, and the result of these efforts is an outcome such as a person's health, morale, or well being.

In the Moos (1980) model, the environmental system includes factors such as the physical design of the setting, the organizational structure, the characteristics of the residents and staff, and the quality of interpersonal relationships. The personal system includes an individual's sociodemographic characteristics and an individual's resources such as health status, cognitive and functional ability, self-esteem, and problem-solving skills.

Cognitive appraisal and coping processes mediate the person–environment transactions. These mediating factors emphasize the active participation of residents in choosing those aspects of the environment to which they will respond. A resident, for example, may or may not choose to participate in a social activity, and participation may or may not increase their morale and or well-being.

Efforts at adaptation affect outcome indices such as the resident's health, well being, and level of functioning. These outcome criteria may also be affected by personal factors (e.g., residents with higher functional ability on admission usually function better six months later) and environmental factors (e.g., facilities with more opportunity for choice tend to have residents with higher morale) (Moos & Lemke, 1985).

NURSING RESEARCH ON ENVIRONMENT AND AGING

In reviewing the research on "Environment and Aging," two important observations were made. One, although the key concepts in most nursing theories are individual, society, health, nursing, and environment (Fawcett, 1983), there has been relatively little research on the environment of health care facilities by nurses. This is of particular interest in view of the fact that in Florence Nightingale's book, *Notes on Nursing: What It Is and What It Is Not* (1859, 1980), eight of the thirteen chapters deal exclusively with the environment.

Most nursing research on the environment has examined the effects of noise levels in intensive care units, recovery rooms, and acute-care wards (Aiken, 1982; Hilton, 1985; Minckley, 1968; Topf, 1984; Woods & Falk, 1974). There

Figure 1

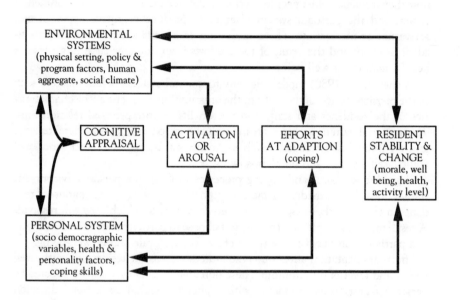

From Moos, R.H. (1980). Specialized living environments for older people: A conceptual framework for evaluation. *Journal of Social Issues*, 36(2), 75–96.

is a small body of research in long-term care focusing on the modification of the environment for the cognitively and chronically-ill patient (Andreasen, 1985; El-Sherif, 1986; Hatton, 1977; Hayter, 1983; Ryden, 1985), the effects of white uniforms on visually and cognitively impaired older patients (Steffes & Thralow, 1985), and on patients' wishes regarding type of room accommodation (Kayser-Jones, 1986). Williams (1988) has recently done a thorough review of research on the physical environment and patient care.

Second, although there are some limitations in environmental research studies in terms of methodology and the lack of a clear theoretical framework, the disparity between what is known about the importance of the environment in promoting well being in long-term care institutions, and what one finds in practice is enormous.

THE IMPORTANCE OF THE ENVIRONMENT IN THE CARE OF THE INSTITUTIONALIZED AGED

Using data from three research projects, I will illustrate the importance of the environment in providing quality care to the institutionalized elderly. First, I will present data to explain the importance of the physical environment. Second, I will focus on the significance of the psychosocial environment. Third, I will present data illustrating the importance of the organizational climate of a skilled nursing facility. Although I will present each part separately, I must emphasize that these components (physical, psychosocial, and organizational) along with the personal environment, are in constant interaction with, and thus influence, one another.

The Physical Environment

My interest in the environmental needs of the elderly dates from a research project that I conducted in 1975 while a doctoral student at the University of California at Berkeley. While conducting research in a nursing home, it came to my attention that many of the residents once they entered the nursing home never left the building. Furthermore, from the window in their rooms, most residents could see only the concrete walls of the adjacent building. They could not see flowers, trees, birds, or clouds in the sky.

In 1977, I conducted a cross-cultural study of one long-term care facility in Scotland and one in the United States. I was struck by the difference in the two environments. The American nursing home, although modern and pleasant in some respects, had an oppressive and institutional atmosphere. By comparison, the Scottish nursing home, a building that was over 100 years old and in many ways physically inconvenient, was more cheerful and homey (Kayser-Jones, 1981, 1981a, 1982).

Research on Room Accommodations. Four years later, I was asked to design a research project to evaluate the quality of care and resident satisfaction or dissatisfaction with care in a 1,270 bed government owned long-term care facility (LTC) that had been built in 1926 (Kayser-Jones, 1986).

This facility was owned and operated by the city and county through the Department of Public Health. It was one of the few remaining publicly owned long-term care facilities in the state, and it was the only institution in the city that readily accepted Medicaid patients requiring skilled nursing care. Therefore, it served as the major provider of LTC services to the indigent elderly in this city.

Over the years, the hospital had been faced with a serious problem concerning its Medicaid certification; it did not meet a federal regulation that stated: "rooms must not contain more than four beds" (Federal Register, 1980). The residents at the hospital were housed in two buildings: a large 1,100-bed facility and a smaller 170-bed building.

The large building contained 30 units; each unit housed 30 residents in open ward accommodations similar to the Nightingale wards in British hospitals, and there were a few private and semiprivate rooms on each unit. The city remodeled the smaller building converting the wards into private, semiprivate, three- and four-bed rooms to comply with the federal regulation. It was opened in January 1981, and gradually residents were transferred from the large to the renovated building.

Before making a decision about the future of the 1,100-bed building, city officials wished to study the situation, and I was asked to design a proposal to evaluate the quality of care at the facility.

The purpose of the research was to compare the quality of care and resident satisfaction or dissatisfaction with care for like groups of residents on the open wards in the large building and in semiprivate rooms in the renovated building. The study used two research strategies: a quantitative study using a validated set of instruments called the "Quality Evaluation System" and an anthropological field study using participant observation and in-depth interviews to obtain qualitative data.

Findings. A major finding of this research was that there was no significant difference in the quality of care on the open wards and in semiprivate rooms.

The most interesting finding to emerge was the response to the question on type of room accommodation preferred. Of the 50 residents on the open ward who were interviewed, 44 (88 percent) said they preferred the open ward to any other type of room accommodation, four residents (8 percent) preferred a private room, and 2 (4 percent) preferred a two-bed room.

The residents who preferred a two-bed room were a man and woman who had become close friends and wanted a room together. The four residents who preferred a private room were relatively young: 33, 40, 51, and 63 years of age. These respondents wanted privacy for entertaining visitors and a quiet place to read, away from the noise of the ward. The open wards, however, were clearly advantageous to the elderly residents for the following reasons.

Advantages of the open ward. First, residents on the open ward said they felt less lonely, isolated, and alone. A private room, they said, would be too lonely. "I want to share my life with someone," observed one man. "Loneliness is a hazard; it is a hazard not to have friends," said another.

Second, residents said they preferred the open ward to a semiprivate room because they feared being placed in a room with an incompatible roommate. On the open ward they could avoid those with whom they did not wish to associate; in a two-bed room, there was no escape.

Third, 60 percent of the respondents indicated that the open wards were an important source of sensory and psychosocial stimulation. Residents with poor vision commented that since they could not see, they enjoyed hearing other people around them, and those with severe hearing losses said they enjoyed watching the activity of others.

Seventy-four percent of the residents were wheelchair bound; they preferred the open ward because they liked to be in a busy, active environment. "If you are dependent on other people to get you around, it is better to be in the middle of everything," observed an immobile woman. Even residents who were not functionally impaired spoke of the psychosocial advantages of the open ward. "I like to be in a group," one woman said. "You have to have friends; we live longer when we can talk with each other." I observed that many patients on the open wards were supportive of and helpful to one another. The less impaired were protective of those residents who were severely disabled. Patients noted that concern for others tended to take their minds off personal problems, and this concern added meaning to their lives.

Fourth, the wards were like small communities with a unique social organization where friendships and conflicts developed, and where people shared goods and services. I learned serendipitously, for example, that informal support groups among visitors had developed on some of the wards. The support that visitors gave to one another was invaluable. One woman who had visited her aphasic, mentally impaired husband twice a day for the past nine years said she could not have endured had it not been for the support of other visitors.

Disadvantages of the open ward. On the other hand, there were some disadvantages to the open ward. Some residents had difficulty sleeping because of the noise on the ward, and others confided that integrating the confused with the alert residents annoyed those who were mentally unimpaired. And there were a few residents who said they valued, needed, and wanted the privacy of a single room.

I want to emphasize that I am not advocating the warehousing of elderly people by placing them in large open wards to reduce the cost of long-term care. Warehousing of the elderly can and does occur in modern facilities that have only private and semiprivate rooms, and it can also occur in institutions with open wards.

It is important for policymakers, health care professionals, and others involved in planning and providing long-term care to recognize that the type of room accommodation is but one factor in determining the quality of care; there are other factors that are also essential.

First, the administrative and professional leadership and the philosophy of care is a critical factor. While the physical structure of a building is important, it is the people, especially the staff, who determine the quality of care. The administrative staff in this facility was progressive, patient oriented, and open to and supportive of creative and innovative ideas. There was strong consistent nursing leadership by the director of nursing, and nursing salaries were competitive. Staff turnover was, therefore, much lower than in most nursing homes.

Second, the activities and services that an institution provides are of paramount importance. The activity department provided interesting and meaningful recreation for the residents; every day, for example, busloads of residents were taken for outings. Furthermore, residents could take photography and art classes, work in a greenhouse, and they had access to a large library.

Third, while conducting this research, I began to appreciate the importance of the institutional milieu in providing quality patient care. While doing participant observation, I observed that the architectural design of the large building and the resources it provided were important factors that contributed to the residents' satisfaction with care.

The large building was a thriving, fascinating place, similar in many ways to a small village. Within the physical structure of the building there was a theater, library, chapel, cafeteria, garden shop, snack shop, small boutique, photography club, and a private kitchen and dining room that could be reserved by residents who wanted to have dinner with friends or relatives. The old large building offered many amenities that made it an attractive environment. It provided residents with an opportunity for choices and allowed them to feel they were part of a vibrant community. On one occasion, for example, I observed an elderly woman sitting on a bench along a corridor; she was wearing a hat and carrying a handbag. I asked where she was going. "Shopping," she replied. She was enroute to the boutique to buy a new sweater.

The renovated building although beautiful, clean, and modern was cold and sterile. The patients called it the "Ice Palace." One woman said she had been taken on a tour of the renovated building, but she did not want to move there. "It's clean, but it is so lonely. There is not a soul sitting in the halls. It is like a mausoleum," she said.

Areas Accessible to Residents in Long-Term Care Institutions. Most long-term care institutions have four or five specific areas where residents spend most of their time: a foyer, the bedroom, the corridor, and a lounge/dining room. Since most nursing home residents do not leave the facility on a regular basis, and many will spend the rest of their lives there, the architectural design and decor of these areas is very important.

Foyer. The foyer in the old large building was a favorite place for many residents who liked to sit there and watch people come and go. The chairs in the foyer were a bright orange color, and there were colorful mosaic tiles and beautifully painted murals on the walls. At all hours of the day, residents could be found sitting in the foyer reading or visiting with one another.

In contrast, residents were seldom seen sitting in the foyer of the renovated building. There were a few chairs lining the bare white walls. There were no paintings on the walls and no plants in the foyer; there were none of the amenities that would make it a pleasant place for residents to congregate.

Bedrooms. Many authorities in the field of environmental research feel that most nursing home residents should be accommodated in private rooms. Koncelik (1976) believes that to have autonomy and to gain control of the space, the resident must be the only inhabitant in the room.

The data from this research disclosed that while there should be some private rooms for those who want complete privacy, residents in the multibed wards, in some respects, had more autonomy and control than residents in the private and semiprivate rooms in the renovated building. We observed, for example, that when residents on the open ward needed a bedpan, there was nearly always a nurse nearby, and they could merely ask for the bedpan. If the nurse ignored this request, another resident might go to their aid and insist that the nurse give them the bedpan. By comparison, residents in the private and semiprivate rooms stated that often they had to wait an hour or longer for someone to bring them a bedpan. They could put on their call light, but if the nursing staff chose to ignore the light, they were unable to do anything more.

We also observed that the open wards had unique personalities. Some of the wards were painted a soft golden color, giving them a feeling of warmth, while others were painted a cool blue-green color, conveying a cold feeling. In some of the wards, there were flowers, plants, and paintings on the walls, while in other wards the walls were bare.

The head nurse on a heavy care ward, while perhaps not theoretically aware of the importance of the environment in providing quality care, had in fact created a splendid environment for the residents. The patients on this ward were severely impaired, physically and mentally. The head nurse had become very attached to them and had hand knit an afghan for each of them, thus personalizing their environment and giving a homey feeling to the ward. Furthermore, despite their level of impairment, she recognized the importance of sensory and psychosocial stimulation. Parties on the ward during the holidays and on other festive occasions were seen as an important part of patient care. For these occasions, the wards were beautifully decorated; the tables were set with table-cloths and flowers, special food was catered, and the staff joined the residents for lunch or refreshments, thus promoting a social rather than a strictly professional relationship.

Church services also were held on some of the wards. In a particularly touching scene, we observed a resident with severe mental impairment begin to cry as the staff and the priest sang "Ave Maria." Although the patient was unable to say what the music meant to her, undoubtedly it was of special significance.

As mentioned above, many of the residents said they did not want to be alone. We often found residents sitting at their bedside engaged in a solitary activity. Each was doing something privately, yet they were not alone.

The residents also informed us that they liked having the nurses nearby; on the open ward, during most of their waking hours the nurses were within their view. Having the nursing staff nearby gave them a sense of security, and the bond between residents and nursing staff was strong. James and Tatton-Brown (1986) in a recently published book on hospital design, note that patients are less concerned with their material surroundings than with seeing and hearing the people who provide their care. Furthermore, residents are more tolerant of delay when calling a nurse if they can see the nurse helping a patient at the other end of the ward, knowing that another patient is in greater need.

In the renovated building, which contained private, semiprivate, three- and four-bed rooms, the bare walls were painted white. A great deal of money had been spent during the renovation, and a policy had been established forbidding patients to place any items on the wall. Due to the lack of color and personal items, the rooms were cold and institutional.

In her book, *Notes on Nursing* (1859, 1980), Florence Nightingale said: "The effect on sickness of beautiful objects, of variety of objects, and especially of brilliancy of color is hardly at all appreciated." The same walls, the same ceiling, were known to make "nerves of the sick suffer." She emphasized that variety from hanging different pictures or by adding bouquets of flowers was a stimulus for patients to take their minds off their suffering.

When renovating the smaller building, strict fire codes had to be adhered to. The fire code mandated that heavy metal fire doors be placed in the doorways of the patients' rooms, and that they should be closed at all times. The doors were so heavy that many of the elderly residents, especially those with arthritic hands, could not easily open them. Residents were, therefore, virtually imprisoned in their rooms and isolated from the nursing staff.

Our data disclosed that privacy was more of a problem in a two-bed room than in the 30-bed ward. Residents in the semiprivate rooms noted that when one person had a visitor the other person inevitably heard the conversation. Resident incompatibility was a frequent complaint. Complaints centered around one wanting the window open while the other wanted the window closed, one resident wanting to smoke while the other could not tolerate smoking, and one roommate wanting the television on while the other wanted it off. Patients were much more territorial and possessive of their space in the semiprivate room than in the open ward.

In the renovated building, the charge nurses complained that they had difficulty finding the auxillary staff. Whereas on the open ward, the nursing staff was always visible, in the private and semiprivate rooms, staff could slip into a room and watch television out of view of their supervisor.

Corridors. Corridors are an important part of a long-term care facility, and they have desirable or undesirable effects on behavior and communication.

The corridors in the large old building were wide and spacious, enabling people with wheelchairs and walkers to move about easily. There were plants in windowboxes along the corridor, paintings done by residents hung on the walls, sunlight streamed in from the windows, and tables and chairs were placed strategically along the hallways so that residents could congregate as they liked. One of the most important features of the hallways in the large building were the sizable windows which enabled the residents to look out and enjoy nature, an important feature for people who have to spend most of their time indoors.

In the large building, there was nearly always someone in the corridor. Alexander, Ishikawa, and Silverstein (1977) note that corridors must have windows so that people can look out. If a corridor does not have windows, they note, people will not want to spend time there.

Privacy is important, and every institution should have some areas where residents can have privacy. In the large building, there were many nooks and crannies where residents could find a private space; residents were often seen sitting quietly by a window in the corridor, looking out of the window or reading a book. Some residents always could be found in a favorite place. One man, for example, could see the ocean from one of the windows in the hallway; every day he sat by the window looking out at the ocean.

Whereas the corridors in the old building were bright, colorful, alive, and often filled with staff, residents, and visitors, the hallways in the renovated building were windowless (for the most part), cold, dark, and devoid of people.

Similar to the bedrooms, the walls of the corridors in the renovated building were painted white; the floors were covered with a light, shiny gray tile. The walls and the floors joined without a distinguishable edge. When this occurs, patients with visual impairment are more likely to bump into the walls and injure themselves. The walls and the floors had a reflective, glossy surface, making the floors appear shiny and slippery. Although one cannot be absolutely certain about the effect this has on behavior, we can be reasonably certain that residents with visual, hearing, and mobility problems would be fearful of falling when walking in such a hallway. Such an environment, therefore, discourages ambulation.

In the renovated building, while standing at one end of the corridor, the long unvarying, windowless hallway produced a dark tunnel-like effect. To add to the problem, there were no chairs for residents to sit on if they needed a brief rest while walking from one end to the other. Residents were sometimes seen leaning against the wall, attempting to rest for a few moments before moving on.

Nursing home residents would often rather be in the corridors than in the lounge. If hallways are not designed to provide small areas for socializing, residents have no choice but to meet in the lounge, which is usually large, noisy, and not conducive to socialization. Furthermore, if hallways do not provide space for residents to stop and rest, falls are more likely to occur.

Lounges. One of the biggest mistakes made in building nursing homes in this country is that typical nursing homes have one large room that serves as a lounge/dining room, and it is usually the only place in the facility where residents and their families can socialize. These lounges are the result of regulations specifying that a certain number of square feet must be provided for each bed (Koncelik, 1976). These multifunctional lounges are usually loud and noisy; thus, they do not provide an environment conducive to relaxation. Several small lounges, a dining room, and perhaps a television room, so that residents could congregate in small groups, would promote socialization and give residents some choice as to where they spend their time.

In the large old building, there were no rooms designated as lounges. The corridors, however, were spacious and small lounges were created in various convenient locations. Furthermore, the long corridors were broken up at intervals by alcoves. These alcoves functioned as small lounges and provided an ideal place for group activities.

By comparison, the renovated building had one huge lounge to accommodate the 170 residents. Although the chairs in the room were a warm orange color, the room appeared sterile and cold. The chairs were placed around the periphery of the room, usually in a straight row, making conversation difficult. There were some small round tables and chairs placed toward the center of the room, but residents seldom sat at these tables. When sitting at these tables, there was the feeling of being "on stage," which discouraged their use. Even during Christmas, with a Christmas tree and other decorations in the lounge, the room did not appear warm and festive.

The large lounge did not promote social interaction. During my observations, I seldom saw people engaged in conversation. On one occasion, I sat in the room for one hour; during that time, only four people spoke to one another. This lounge provided a perfect example of how poor architectural design can create an environment that has a negative effect on behavior.

Dining room. Nursing homes are required to have a dining room so that socialization will occur at mealtime. Although in the renovated building the staff put a great deal of thought into decorating the dining room, it was something of a failure. The dining room was furnished with small tables accommodating four to six residents. However, one seldom observed residents talking with one another.

While nicely decorated, the dining room was large. Carts with the food trays were wheeled into the dining room, producing a great deal of noise and confusion at mealtime. The food was served in compartmentalized plastic trays. Prior to the renovation, the food was served on china plates. The residents did not enjoy eating off of plastic trays. The coffee cups were covered with loose plastic. Since the food was transported a long distance from the old building, the coffee often spilled onto the food, making it unattractive and unappealing. Interestingly, despite a nicely decorated dining room, there were more complaints about the food in the new building than in the old one.

The Psychosocial Environment

I have been emphasizing the physical features of the environment, which are critically important. No less important, however, are the psychosocial components.

Koncelik (1976) notes that in the rush to improve the more glaring faults of institutional care, the less tangible elements were left undeveloped. For example, the sterile and clinical atmosphere of many nursing homes, the lack of individuality in room decor, the high noise levels in some nursing homes and the deafening silence in others, the offensive odors, and the unpleasant sounds undoubtedly have an impact on the quality of life of nursing home residents.

The importance of sensory stimulation for the normal development of perceptual and cognitive functions as well as for the maintenance of normal behavior has been well documented (Wohlwill, 1966). Much of the research in this area has focused on the harmful effects of drastic reductions in levels of stimulation. For example, the research on the effects of sensory deprivation is unequivocal (Zubek, 1969). Despite the availability of these research findings, however, many nursing home residents receive minimal sensory stimulation.

This is especially true for patients with impaired vision and hearing. A few years ago I was asked to present a paper on the consequences of hearing impairment for nursing home residents. I designed a small study to investigate the consequences of hearing impairment for the institutionalized elderly. I went to a skilled nursing facility and asked the staff for a list of hearing-impaired residents whom I could interview. Mr. T., I was told, had a severe hearing loss. I walked into his room and found a man apathetic and withdrawn, lying in bed, looking at a blank white wall before him. I spoke with him and learned after only a few moments that he was an opera singer with an international reputation. This man, whose entire life had been devoted to opera, had no access to music.

Mr. T. had been born in Wales, the son of a coal miner; his father had died in a mining accident before he was born. My husband is British and traces his ancestry to Wales. Therefore, we have some beautiful Welsh music on records, and when I told my husband about this man, he arranged to have the music from the records transferred to a tape.

We took the tape and a tape player with stereo headphones to the nursing home so that Mr. T. could once again hear some music. We placed the earphones on his ears and turned on the tape player, not knowing if he would be able to hear because of his severe hearing impairment. As the music began to play, his eyes widened in surprise and tears began to flow down his cheeks as he listened to the beautiful music from his homeland.

This was a very successful and rewarding experience, and we became involved with this man and anxious to see what other type of sensory stimulation we could provide. His wife told us that his favorite opera was I Pagliacci. Therefore, we obtained a tape of the opera and returned to the nursing home.

First, we showed him the tape; he expressed interest in the picture on the box. As the music began to play, his face became animated and joyful and his eyes danced with excitement and pleasure.

His wife became enthusiastic about his obvious response to and enjoyment of this sensory stimulation and decided to bring in photographs of Mr. T. in some of his opera costumes. She placed the photographs on the wall opposite his bed. The nursing staff was fascinated when they learned of Mr. T.'s past achievements and decided that it would be a good idea to organize group sessions for the purpose of learning something of the other residents' past lives.

This experience was a powerful example of how one can change the psychosocial environment of a nursing home resident. This man came to life before our eyes, and there is no doubt that the music we provided contributed greatly to the quality of his life during his last few months. I was amazed that the nursing staff knew so little about the past history of their residents, and I began to reflect upon the organizational features of the environment that allows such neglect to happen.

The Organizational Features of the Environment

A current research project designed to investigate the social and cultural factors that influence the decision-making process when nursing home residents acquire an acute illness will illustrate the importance of the organizational components of the environment. While conducting this research, 100 nursing home residents, family members, doctors, and nursing staff (a total of 400 subjects) were interviewed. We also followed 215 residents, describing in detail exactly what happened when they developed an acute illness. Data were collected in three skilled nursing facilities.

When analyzing our data, we found that in some cases acute illnesses occurred because of organizational factors that contributed to poor nursing care. To reiterate, the organizational climate includes items such as policy, staffing, and financing of health care. Policy issues and an inadequate number of competent professional and paraprofessional staff were the major organizational problems.

For example, the implementation of a major new health policy, diagnosis related groups (DRGs), has affected the quality of care in nursing homes. During the course of the research, we observed that there was an increasingly large number of heavy care patients in the nursing homes. To confirm our observations, we asked the charge nurse on one unit if they were admitting more patients who where in a subacute rather than in a chronic condition. "Yes," she replied, "we are and I don't like it. The aides aren't able to handle these patients." The hospitals are discharging patients earlier, but the nursing homes are not increasing their professional or nonprofessional staff to provide the necessary care.

On one occasion, a patient was admitted to the nursing home with a tracheostomy. I asked the geriatric nurse practitioner if they were able to provide adequate nursing care to this patient. "No," she said. "She should be suctioned every hour, but she will be lucky if she gets suctioned once a shift." This same nurse confided that even patients who are receiving antibiotics for pneumonia may not recover because no one has the time to encourage them to cough and deep breathe every few hours.

Nutritional Problems.   Adequate nutrition for the elderly depends upon multiple physical, psychological, and environmental factors. Nightingale (1859, 1980) in her book, *Notes on Nursing,* said: "Every careful observer of the sick will agree in this that thousands of patients are annually starved in the midst of plenty from want of attention to the ways which alone make it possible for them to take food."

Florence Nightingale wrote that statement in 1859; it is shocking that 130 years later patients in nursing homes are suffering from poor nutrition and dehydration due to environmental factors.

In our study, we did not ask residents their opinions about the food. At the end of the interview, however, we did ask: "How do you feel about your life here in the nursing home?" For example, "Are you happy with your care?"

In response to this question, food was frequently the first concern mentioned. Many of the residents were dissatisfied with their meals; only two made favorable comments about the food.

Complaints about food centered around three issues: (1) the unpleasant features of the dining room; (2) the manner in which meals were served; and (3) the poor quality of the food.

The unpleasant features of the dining room. Nursing homes are required to have an area designated for eating because dining rooms supposedly will contribute to socialization and make mealtime a pleasant social experience. The residents reported, however, that the dining room was noisy, crowded, and in general an unpleasant atmosphere. Staff shouted back and forth to one another during mealtime. The mentally impaired residents often cried out incoherently. One woman called loudly, "mama, mama," was silent momentarily and then began to call again. Since there was only one dining room, the mentally impaired residents ate with those who were unimpaired. It was unpleasant for the mentally alert to observe others as they spilled food on themselves while attempting to eat. No effort was made to seat residents at tables according to their social preference and their manipulative ability to handle food.

Noise. Due to the noise in the dining room and the lack of effort to seat residents who could socialize with one another at one table, there was virtually no conversation during mealtime.

The unpleasant atmosphere of the dining room did not promote good nutrition. An 83-year-old mentally alert woman vividly described an especially distasteful experience. When she went to the dining room to eat, she was placed beside a man whose urinal was hanging on the side of his wheelchair. There was urine in the urinal, and she found the odor offensive. This woman was shocked and upset when the man used the urinal again while in the dining room. His behavior was so objectional that she fictitiously told the nurse she had to go to the bathroom immediately so that she could leave the dining room. "That was my last time in the dining room," she said. "I eat better alone in my room."

Manner in which food is served. The manner in which food was served (due primarily to a shortage of nursing staff) also contributed to poor nutritional intake. Meals were served in a task-oriented, hurried manner. The nurses remarked that they had to rush to serve the food and feed patients in a short period of time before the kitchen staff came to remove the trays. In one facility, patients who had to be fed were placed at one end of the dining room; one nurse aide was responsible for feeding five to six residents simultaneously. She rushed back and forth among them, grateful for those who ate quickly.

Residents who were not totally dependent but who needed some assistance with eating were perhaps the most disadvantaged. A frail, emaciated man with Parkinson's disease struggled slowly and laboriously to feed himself. Most of the food fell from the trembling fork before it reached his mouth. A research assistant was concerned that they would take the tray away before he had finished his meal and asked the staff if they would like her to assist him. The nurse aide informed her that he was not a "feeder." This case illustrates how a physical/ functional disability combined with an environmental constraint contributes to nutritional problems.

To expedite the feeding of patients, some staff members mixed all of the food together. One woman commented upon how distasteful it was to have to observe patients eat in this way.

One man who could eat independently complained about the manner in which meals were served. "Meal times are bad," he said. "They stuff food in your mouth. Patients are treated carelessly here. Feeding is a big problem. They take the food away before you are finished. If we could just be treated like we would be in a restaurant where you can finish your food. They should feed patients slowly," he continued. "I don't like to eat fast. You get patients well by feeding them; the doctors want that."

Quality of food. Throughout the study, we had made general observations about the food with the hypothesis in mind that poor nutrition might contribute to an acute illness. Although we had significant objective data on the subject of food, I decided to observe the residents and staff throughout an entire mealtime. It was one of the most powerful experiences I have ever had!

I went to the dining room shortly after trays had been served. It was a depressing scene. I was shocked and saddened to find that eating, which for most of us is a pleasant, enjoyable event could be reduced to an almost subhuman level.

Five or six patients were sitting at two large round tables. There were no tablecloths, place mats, or flowers on the tables. A television with the evening news provided the only sound of voices in the dining room.

About half of the residents, apparently those with teeth, had soup, a liverwurst sandwich, a brownie, fruit cocktail, and tea, coffee or milk. Many of the patients had only pureed food. The pureed food was served in a round, compartmentalized plastic dish. In one compartment were mashed potatoes; a thin dark brown substance (apparently pureed meat), and a watery yellowish substance, which I assumed was pureed carrots, were in the other two sections of the dish.

One woman was attempting to eat the food with a fork, but except for the mashed potatoes, which were of the proper consistency, all of the other food was so thin that it ran through the tines of the fork, onto her chin, down the front of her clothing, and onto the tray and table. A man with a severe tremor of his hands spilled coffee on his sandwich as he attempted to drink independently. Others struggled to eat as best they could.

Data from the family interviews confirmed our observations that due to staffing deficiencies, many patients who needed help with eating were left unaided. A family member said, "The staff say the patients won't eat, but they leave the tray and don't help him, and he is weak. They don't have time to feed him. They come in and if they can't shovel it in, it is all over. They just take it away. When I feed him, it takes almost an hour."

In analyzing data from acute illness episodes, we found that several residents who were sent to the hospital in an acute condition were found to be severely dehydrated. A 102-year-old ambulatory woman was admitted to the nursing home on the first of the month weighing 114 pounds. She had trouble swallowing, and she had a tendency to put too much food in her mouth which precipitated choking. Twenty days later she had lost 22 pounds, and then weighed a mere 92 pounds. She was admitted to the acute hospital with a diagnosis of pneumonia and dehydration. The attending physician reported that this woman was so dehydrated that when she examined her, the patient's tongue was stuck to the roof of her mouth.

Using the case of Mr. T. (the man with hearing impairment) and the 102-year-old woman who became severely dehydrated, I would like to illustrate how the interaction of the various components of the environment affect patient well being (see Figure 1).

In the case of Mr. T., various factors in the environmental system (e.g., staffing levels and lack of professional nursing staff who understand the importance of sensory stimulation) combined with factors from the personal system (hearing and cognitive impairment) interacted to hinder his ability to respond and adapt to a situation which ultimately resulted in a decline in morale and decreased well being.

In the case of the 102-year-old woman, factors from the environmental system (e.g., nursing staff who did not identify the problem she had with eating and inattention to intake and output and weight loss) interacted with factors from the personal system (cognitive impairment, difficulty in swallowing, and no family or friends to intervene on her behalf). According to Moos & Lemke (1985), cognitive appraisal and coping processes mediate the person–environment transactions. In this case, this woman's coping ability was limited due to functional and cognitive impairment; the outcome was a severe weight loss, dehydration, and pneumonia.

CONCLUSION

It is alarming that a basic need such as fluids and nutrition can be so neglected when caring for elderly patients. Dennis & Prescott (1985) found when asking nurses around the country to describe good nursing practice that dietary concerns were not commonly identified as an activity comprising good nursing.

Kayser-Jones (1981) found, when comparing the quality of care in a Scottish and an American institution, that the greatest difference between the two facilities was the environment. In the Scottish institution, the environment was patient centered while, in the American institution, little attempt was made to consider the needs of the elderly residents (Andreasen, 1985).

To provide quality care to the elderly, the nurse must be involved in all aspects of the environment—the physical, the organizational, the personal, and the psychosocial milieu. While all components are important, the nurse's involvement in the organizational aspects of long-term care facilities is essential for quality nursing care. Florence Nightingale emphasized that the nature of the hospital authority (e.g., policy issues) was critical. "For unless an understanding is come to on this point, the very existence of good nursing is an impossibility" (Nightingale, 1859, 1980).

There are many environmental factors that will promote well being for the institutionalized elderly, such as color, lighting, the physical arrangement of furniture, personal belongings, the administrative philosophy, and the absence of irritating noises. Nothing, however, is more important than the characteristics of the nursing staff. Human relationships—the bond between nurse and patient—

are more important than the physical surroundings. Nurses must be involved in planning an environment that will promote and enhance the nurse–patient relationship. Furthermore, we must emphasize the value of the nurse–patient contact and be involved in the design of facilities and the development of policies that will increase this contact and promote the development and maintenance of a strong nurse–patient bond.

REFERENCES

Aiken, R.J. (1982). Quantitative noise analysis in a modern hospital. *Archives of Environmental Health, 37*(6), 361–364.

Alexander, C., Ishikawa, S., & Silverstein, M. (1977). *A Pattern Language: Towns, Buildings, Construction.* New York: Oxford University Press.

Andreasen, M.E. (1985). Make a safe environment by design. *Journal of Gerontological Nursing, 11*(6), 18–22.

Dennis, K.E., & Prescott, P.A. (1985, January). Florence Nightingale: Yesterday, today, and tomorrow. *Advances in Nursing Science,* (pp. 66–81).

El-Sherif, C. (1986, May/June). A unit for the acutely ill. *Geriatric Nursing,* (pp. 130–139).

Fawcett, J. (1983). Hallmarks of success in nursing theory development. In P.L. Chinn (Ed.), *Advances in Nursing Theory Development,* (pp. 3–17). Rockville, MD: Aspen.

Federal Register. (1980). *Conditions of participation for skilled nursing and intermediate care facilities, Part III.* (Department of Health and Human Services, Health Care Financing Administration, 45, 473–482). Baltimore, MD.

Hatton, J. (1977). Aging and the glare problem. *Journal of Gerontological Nursing, 3,* 38–44.

Hayter, J. (1983). Modifying the environment to help older persons. *Nursing & Health Care, 4*(5), 265–269.

Hilton, B.A. (1985). Noise in acute patient care areas. *Research in Nursing and Health, 8,* 283–291.

James, W.P., & Tatton-Brown, W. (1986). *Hospitals: Design and development.* New York: Van Nostrand Reinhold Co., Inc.

Kahana, E. (1982). A congruence model of person-environment interaction. In M.P. Lawton, P.G. Windley, & T.O. Byerts (Eds.), *Aging and the environmental theoretical approaches* (pp. 97–121).

Kahana, E. (1974). Matching environments to needs of the aged: A conceptual scheme. In J.F. Gubrium (Ed.), *Late life: Communities and environmental policy.* Springfield, IL: Charles C. Thomas.

Kayser-Jones, J.S. (1981). *Old, alone, and neglected: Care of the aged in Scotland and the United States.* Berkeley, CA: University of California Press.

Kayser-Jones, J.S. (1981a). A comparison of care in a Scottish and a United States facility. *Geriatric Nursing: American Journal of Care for the Aging, 2*(1), 44–50.

Kayser-Jones, J.S. (1982). Institutional structures: Catalysts of or barriers to quality care for the institutionalized aged in Scotland and the United States. *Social Science and Medicine, 16*(9), 935–944.

Kayser-Jones, J.S. (1986). Open-ward accommodations in a long-term care facility: The elderly's point of view. *The Gerontologist, 26*(1), 63–69.

Koncelik, J.A. (1976). *Designing the open nursing home.* Stroudsburg, PA: Dowden, Hutchinson, & Ross, Inc.

Lawton, M.P. (1975). Competence, environmental press, and adaptation. In P.G. Windley, T.O. Byerts, & G. Ernst (Eds.), *Theory development in environment and aging.* Washington, DC: Gerontological Society.

Lawton, M.P. (1982). Competence, environmental press, and the adaptation of older people. In M.P. Lawton, P.G. Windley, & T.O. Byerts (Eds.), *Aging and the environment: Theoretical approaches* (pp. 33–59). New York: Springer.

Lawton, M.P., & Nahemow, L. (1973). Ecology and the aging process. In C. Eisdorfer & M.P. Lawton (Eds.), *The psychology of adult development and aging.* Washington, DC: American Psychological Association.

Lindheim, R. & Syme, S.L. (1983). Environments, people, and health. *Annual Review Public Health, 4*, 335–359.

Minckley, B.B. (1968). The study of noise and its relationship to patient discomfort in the recovery room. *Nursing Research, 17*(3), 247–250.

Moos, R.H. (1980). Specialized living environments for older people: A conceptual framework for evaluation. *Journal of Social Issues, 36*(2), 75–96.

Moos, R.H., & Lemke, S. (1985). Assessing and improving social-ecological settings. In E. Seidman (Ed.), *Handbook of social intervention.* Beverly Hills, CA: Sage Publications.

Nightingale, F. (1859)(1980). *Notes on nursing: What it is and what it is not.* New York: Churchill Livingstone, Inc.

Ryden, M.B. (1985). Environmental support for autonomy in the institutionalized elderly. *Research in Nursing and Health, 8*, 363–371.

Steffes, R., & Thralow, J. (1985). Do uniform colors keep patients awake? *Journal of Gerontological Nursing, 11*(7), 6–9.

Topf, M. (1984). A framework for research on aversive physical aspects of the environment. *Research in Nursing and Health, 7*, 35–42.

Williams, M.A. (1988). The physical environment and patient care. *Annual Review of Nursing Research, 7*, 61–84.

Woods, N.F., & Falk, S.A. (1974). Noise stimuli in the acute care area. *Nursing Research, 23*(2), 144–150.

Zubek, J.T. (1969). *Sensory deprivation: Fifteen years of research.* New York: Appleton, Century, Croft.

Environment and Quality of Life: A Reaction from the Perspective of Social Science and Environmental Design

Leslie A. Grant, PhD
Research Associate
Institute for Health and Aging
University of California
San Francisco, CA

Dr. Kayser-Jones underscored the importance of environment on quality of life for residents in long-term care institutions. In fact, there is a growing body of research in social gerontology that shows how environment influences adaptation in the aged. Because the environment affects not only how the aged adapt to living in a long-term care facility, but also the overall utilization pattern and need for long-term care and supportive services, it plays a major role.

However, Dr. Kayser-Jones did not directly address another important concern: how the environment outside of long-term care institutions affects quality of life for seniors living in noninstitutional settings. For example, we know that the need for certain types of long-term care services can be eliminated by changes to a person's dwelling unit (Struyk, 1988). Housing modifications such as the installation of grab bars, ramps, specially equiped telephones or other features can compensate for specific functional impairments. The availability of physical amenities also influences the ease with which long-term care services can be provided in the home (Newman, 1985; Noelker, 1982; Soldo & Longino, 1988).

No doubt, a person's living arrangements and the presence of social supports can reduce the risk of nursing home placement (Johnson & Grant, 1985). A Swedish study found that the utilization of hospitals, the number of hospitalizations, and the mean duration of hospital stays are correlated with the size of the dwelling unit (Thiberg, 1988). Elderly who live alone consistently have longer stays in the hospital and fewer discharges than people living together. Many different forms of supportive housing can positively affect the quality of life for seniors and reduce the need for institutionalization (Sherwood, Mor, & Gutkin, 1981; Sherwood & Morris, 1983; Newcomer & Grant, in press). Although it is important to understand how the design of a dwelling unit, living arrangement, and specialized housing contribute to the well being of the noninstitutionalized aged population, the major focus of this reaction will pertain to institutional settings.[1]

Over the years researchers have studied the effects of relocation and institutionalization on long-term care outcomes. In general, researches have found institutional effects to vary depending upon the "totality" of the institution, the personality of the aging individual, and the degree of change or discontinuity between pre- and post-relocation environments. Components of totality which have been studied include the extent of privacy provided, the rigidity of the scheduling and controls, the access to personal property, and the extent of isolation from the outside world (Coe, 1965). The institutional effects common to most types of institutions have been reported by Sommer and Osmond (1961). These effects include deindividuation; disculturation; emotional, social, or physical damage; estrangement; isolation; and stimulus deprivation (Johnson & Grant, 1985).

Studies have shown that the quality of the environment influences successful adaptation of old people relocating to and living in institutional settings (Lieberman & Tobin, 1983; Tobin & Lieberman, 1976). Relocation to the nursing

---

[1] Readers interested in environmental improvements for the frail elderly living in specialized housing and community settings are referred to general reviews by Newcomer, Lawton, and Byerts (1986), Regnier and Pynoos (1987), U.S. Department of Housing and Urban Development (1987), or Committee on an Aging Society (1988). Book chapters and articles about home modifications for the frail elderly are provided by Pynoos et al. (1987), Struyk (1987, 1988), Soldo and Longino (1988), and Moleski (1985).

home frequently occurs at a time when the aging individual has diminished social, psychological, and physical resources. How can the experience of moving into and living in an institution be made less traumatic for the aged?

In this regard, Dr. Kayser-Jones made several major points. Ward design, administrative and professional leadership, philosophy of care, architectural and interior design, the psychosocial milieu, adequate staffing, good dietary practices, and organizational policies are among the critical environmental factors. Human relationships and particularly that bond between patient and nurse are basic to quality of care.

What this paper addresses, then, is not whether the professionalism of the staff is more important to patient outcomes than the physical plant. Both factors are equally vital. A substandard building can be just as life threatening as incompetent nursing staff. In situations where *both* patient care and physical environment are inadequate, the quality of life would be even more seriously jeopardized.

Because the critical issue in the assessment of quality of long-term care services lies ultimately in patient outcomes, this paper will focus on those aspects of the institutional environment critical to long-term care outcomes. First, an overview of current theoretical perspectives on environment, aging, and adaptation is presented. Three general approaches to understanding how the institutional environment affects adaptation in the aged are reviewed: (1) a transactional perspective, (2) a social–ecological perspective, and (3) a person–environment congruence perspective. (These models are summarized in Table 1.) Second, efforts by environmental designers to moderate adverse institutional effects by "deinstitutionalizing" the institution are described.

TRANSACTIONAL MODEL

A transactional model predicts outcomes by looking at the transaction between a person and the environment. Richard Lazarus' (1978) stress and coping paradigm is a transactional model that views the environment from the perspective of cognitive psychology. The relationship between a person and the environment is seen as a dynamic process. Cognitive appraisal and coping mediate this transaction to determine how environmental stressors affect outcomes. A number of studies have been conducted concerning the effects of noxious physical stimuli on behavioral responses or outcomes. For example, heat stress has been linked to responses such as level of arousal, affective states, attention, and perceived control (Bell, 1981). Noise is known to affect human performance,

Table 1
Summary of Major Models of Environment, Aging and Adaptation

Environmental Domain	Personal Domain	Mediating Factors	Outcomes Predicted
Transactional Perspective			
Lazarus' Stress and Coping Paradigm Nonspecific; views environment as a source of stressful stimuli.	Nonspecific; views individual as having differing resources (e.g., psychological, social, or physical) for mastering potentially stressful environmental demands.	Cognitive appraisal and coping.	Nonspecific; a variety of behavioral responses are predicted.
Social–Ecological Perspective			
Moos and Lemke's Multiphasic Environmental Assessment Procedure Environmental resources in four domains: (1) physical and architectural features, (2) policy and program factors, (3) resident and staff characteristics, and (4) social climate.	Individuals in aggregate are viewed as an integral part of the environmental system. Personal system includes sociodemographic variables, roles, expectations, stress, and impairment factors.	Cognitive appraisal, degree of activation, and coping.	Health status and health-related behaviors.
Lawton and Nahemow's Social Ecological Model of Adaptation Personal environment, suprapersonal environment, social environment, and physical environment.	Biological health, sensory–perceptual capacity, motor skills, cognitive capacity, and ego strength are five major areas of	Adaptation level delineates homeostatic balance between environmental press and competence. Outcomes are contingent	Nonspecific; a variety of affective and behavioral outcomes are predicted.

Person–Environment Congruence Perspective

		individual competence.	upon the strength of press relative to competence.	
Kahana's Congruence Model	Segregate dimension, congregate dimension, institutional control, structure, stimulation–engagement, affect, and impulse control.	Parallel personality dimensions (i.e., segregate and congregate dimensions, institutional control, structure, stimulation–engagement, affect and impulse control). Personality dimensions are defined in terms of need or preference.	Degree of congruence of goodness-of-fit between environmental characteristics and individual need or preference.	Life satisfaction and morale.
Lieberman and Tobin's Congruence Model	Achievement fostering, individuation, dependency fostering, warmth, affiliation fostering, recognition, stimulation, physical attractiveness, cue richness, tolerance for deviancy, and health care adequacy.	A person's need for stimulation, achievement, affiliation, autonomy, counteraction, physical maintenance, recognition, and succorance. Personality variables (i.e., activity–passivity, narcissism, aggression, status drive, distrust of others, empathy, extrapunitiveness, intrapunitiveness, authoritarianism–equalitarianism).	Degree of continuity or match between pre- and post-relocation environments. Degree of congruence between traits or needs and environmental qualities.	Short-term stress reactions (i.e., affective, cognitive, behavioral, and social interaction). Long-term adaptive outcomes (i.e., enhanced competency, homeostasis, and adaptive failure).

interpersonal behavior, annoyance, cognitive development, and mental and physical health (Cohen & Weinstein, 1981). In institutional settings, lack of adequate acoustical separation between private and public areas can be a source of discomfort to patients. Adaptive responses to noise are mediated by such things as its predictability, controllability, and meaning. These factors are also known to mediate other types of environmental stress such as that associated with relocation. Other researchers have looked at the effects of crowding, spatial invasion, privacy, territoriality or security on social and psychological functioning (Kaminoff & Proshansky, 1982).

Dr. Kayser-Jones' study about open ward design is a good example of this type. A most intriguing finding of this research concerns open wards. Despite less than optimal environmental conditions, the open wards developed into small communities with unique social organizations. The main building was likened to a "small village" with a variety of amenities and places such as a theater, library, chapel, cafeteria, garden shop, snack shop, and so forth. Unfortunately, however, most nursing homes in the United States provide little else for patients to do than spend their remaining years playing out the sick role attributed to them. All too often the patient role is performed in an institution almost completely given over to medical interventions. With the resulting restriction of social interactions, many older people face the prospect of moving into a nursing home with great fear and apprehension.

Alternatives, however, do exist. For example, create settings that foster the development of patient communities where social roles and group norms extrinsic to the patient role can find expression. In several long-term care institutions which this author has studied, the residents were allowed to have social roles in addition to the patient role, including those of friend, grandparent, elder, nun, helper or leader (Grant, 1982).

Yet in too many institutions social activities have devolved into the "BBCs," that is, bingo, birthday, and crafts. It is important to design physical and social environments in long-term care facilities to maintain the social integration of the patients. The provision of alternative social roles is an important element contributing to quality of life. A valued social role diminishes a person's social isolation and attenuates the "rolelessness" or role loss among the aged living within bounded communities (Rosow, 1967). There is a need to create long-term care settings for the aged that foster the development of resident communities. We will return to the issue of creating viable patient communities later in this paper.

SOCIAL–ECOLOGICAL MODEL

A second type of general theoretical perspective, the social–ecological perspective, views the person, the social environment, and the physical environment as essential components of a general ecological system in which interdependent parts are defined to represent other salient elements of the environmental system. Rudolph Moos' (1980) social–ecological model, which was described by Dr. Kayser-Jones, identifies physical and architectural features, policy and program factors, aggregate resident and staff characteristics, and social climate as components of an overall social–ecological system.

Another social–ecological model developed by Lawton and Nahemow (1973) predicts behavioral outcomes by looking at an individual's "competence" in relation to "environmental press." Competence includes a person's biological health, sensory perceptual capacity, motor skills, cognitive capacity, and ego strength. Adaptation is predicted by examining the fit between competence and the demands of the environment. Environmental press encompasses multiple demands that the environment places upon individuals. These demands include aspects of the physical environment such as ambient temperature, levels and types of lighting, environmental prostheses such as ramps and grab bars, orientational cues, or geographic distance. Outcomes for individuals are dependent upon the strength of enviromental press in relation to an individual's adaptation level and his or her competence. People with high degrees of competence are thought to adapt successfully under higher levels of environmental press. They are believed to be less sensitive than those of low competence to discrepancies between their adaptation level and the environmental press they encounter.

These two social–ecological models differ in terms of *how* the environment is thought to affect outcomes. Moos' (1980) conceptualization draws upon Lazarus' (1978) transactional model. It emphasizes mediating cognitive processes of appraisal and coping to determine outcomes. Lawton and Nahemow's (1973) model predicts adaptation through the specification of optimal relationships between distinct dimensions within the personal and environmental domains. The person, environmental press, and behavioral outcomes are linked through Helson's (1964) concept of adaptation level which refers to the normal homeostatic point where the demands of the environment are approximately equal to an individual's level of competence. This model emphasizes a more homeostatic view of adaptation. Both of these social–ecological models describe a transactional relationship in that each assumes a potentially bidirectional or reciprocal interchange between person and environment.

PERSON–ENVIRONMENT CONGRUENCE MODEL

Person–environment congruence models examine the goodness of fit between a set of personality characteristics and a commensurate set of environmental demands. These models differ from those previously discussed in their focus on the discrepancy between specific dimensions of personality and press or demand in equivalent environmental parameters. Such a discrepancy is seen as a potential source of stress. Kahana's (1982) model predicts outcomes on the basis of the discrepancy between personality and environmental characteristics along seven dimensions which are shown in Table 1. Several studies (Kahana, Liang, & Felton, 1977; Kiyak, 1977) have found that congruence between personality (i.e., personal needs or preferences) and environmental press predict life satisfaction and morale among the institutionalized aged.

Lieberman and Sheldon's (1983) person–environment congruence model looks at personality in relation to 11 environmental dimensions which are also shown in Table 1. These researchers have studied the relationship between environmental change and personality by drawing upon four types of relocation. They found that the most powerful predictors of adaptation were not, as expected, personality factors but three environmental factors: (1) the quality of the new environment, (2) its congruence with the individual's needs, and (3) the extent of continuity with the previous environment.

In summary, a wide rage of conceptual approaches have been developed. All the models reviewed here use the concepts of environmental press or environmental stress to predict individual outcomes. The fundamental difference between "press" and "stress" is that the former is a more neutral term. Press may or may not lead to stress. Equilibrium is maintained within a variable range of environmental press. Stress implies a state of disequilibrium. However, neither term denotes a state that necessarily leads to an adverse outcome for the individual. Salient characteristics of the individual which mediate the person–environment interchange have been described in such terms as cognitive appraisal, coping, competence, adaptation level, personality traits, preference, and need.

In the present context, new theoretical models are needed to articulate what the environmental dimensions relevant to nursing care and what the critical components of the physical and social environments are. Since Dr. Kayser-Jones has already addressed major issues which are relevant to nursing practice, the remainder of this paper will focus on important dimensions of the physical and social environments. The level of analysis will shift from abstract theoretics to applied or practical aspects of designing more optimal environments for long-term institutional care.

ENVIRONMENTAL DESIGN

Architectural problems invariably involve the design of physical environments to satisfy the requirements of human needs and activities. Architects cannot conceive of buildings or communities apart from the human activities they serve. An increasing specialization within architectural practice is occurring due to the historical increase in the number of different building types and their growing complexity. Fitch (1972) estimates that there are now about 300 different kinds of buildings regularly under construction in modern industrial societies, compared to perhaps 25 or so common during the nineteenth century. Gradually, the workability of building design has been redefined to encompass more than just construction and maintenance costs, or the adequacy of lighting, heating, and acoustics in determining the operational criteria for building design. Architects have begun to take greater interest in the impact of the built environment on behavioral outcomes.

Here is an opportunity for collaboration between nurses and architects. Nursing professionals can contribute to the architectural design process by helping the architect to better understand the special needs of the long-term care patient. "Programming" refers to the development of design criteria which is a necessary first step before any building can be designed. It is during the programming phase that nurses can directly assist architects by clarifying the requirements for good patient care.

In designing a long-term care facility, architects are faced with many constraints. Regulatory requirements embodied in state licensure and federal certification standards emphasize life and fire safety. Dimensions enhancing the psychosocial environment are not mandated by law. Where economic constraints are severe, minimum standards in regulations may become maximum standards. This tendency for minimum requisites to set operational limits can affect multiple environmental parameters such as the number of staff per patient, the ratio of professional to nonprofessional staff, the ratio of private to shared rooms, the levels of social amenities provided or the amount of space allocated per bed. In order to create more optimal environments within long-term care facilities, it may be necessary to commit sufficient economic and social resources to exceed the regulatory minimums.

A well-designed long-term care facility must be responsive to the needs of the individual patient. This basic point is illustrated by contrasting several divergent needs between the Alzheimer's patient and the cognitively nonimpaired. An Alzheimer's patient who is coping with memory loss may benefit from living in an environment that is structured, regimented, and predictable. An unpredictable or inconsistent environment (e.g., one that offers constantly changing mealtimes, constant reassignment of caregivers, or other inconsisten-cies in daily routines) may overwhelm someone who is coping with memory loss. An Alzheimer's patient might also benefit from a small unit size which makes it easier to find one's room and facilitates way-finding. On the other hand, for someone who is *not* cognitively impaired, strict regimentation in daily routines may undermine independence and contribute to "learned helplessness," which refers to an inability among some institutionalized persons to make per-sonal decisions due to a loss in personal autonomy. Flexibility in daily routines may allow for greater choice and autonomy in decision making. A larger unit size may present greater opportunities for making new friends or finding compat-ible roommates. It is important for architects to understand what the needs of the users are—be they nursing staff, patients, or their family members.

Deinstitutionalizing the Institution

Environmental designers have attempted to make the experience of moving into and living in a nursing home less traumatic for the elderly. These efforts have focused on modifying the monotonous environment of the nursing home and thereby "deinstitutionalizing" the institutional setting. Designers have made progress toward making the nursing home environment better suited to the special needs of the aged. Innovators in architectural and interior design have sought to create a "total managed environment" wherein social and environmen-tal factors, rather than the medical regimen alone, are subject to intervention. Rather than forcing the individual to adapt to the institution, progress has been made toward modifying the institutional environment and making it more re-sponsive to the needs of the aging individual. Some specific points are illustrated below.

Stimulus deprivation can lead to a deadening of senses in an individual who has grown accustomed to the monotony of the institutional environment. Sen-sory deprivation, heightend by isolation from society at large, can cause a downward spiral of further deterioration (Johnson & Grant, 1985). Reduced sensory acuity in vision and hearing compounds sensory deprivation and also may be a source of confusion in some aged patients. Stimulus deprivation can be minimized by the use of color, natural light, and views. It has been advocated that both color and light be manipulated in the institutional environment to minimize the effects of stimulus deprivation and to enhance mood. Color coding and cueing also can aid in improving functions in self-care and orientation or way-finding (Cooper, Gowland, & McIntosh, 1986).

Age-related changes in vision and hearing often lead to perceptual changes in older patients (Christenson, 1983; Cooper, Gowland, & McIntosh, 1986). A gradual hardening of the lens of the eye reduces its ability to change shape

Lawton, M.P., & Nahemow, L. (1973). Ecology and the aging process. In C. Eisdorfer & M.P. Lawton (Eds.), *The psychology of adult development and aging*. Washington, DC: American Psychological Association.

Lazarus, R. (1978). *The stress and coping paradigm*. Paper presented at The Critical Evaluation of Behavioral Paradigms for Psychiatric Science, Glendon Beach, Oregon.

Lieberman, M., & Tobin, S. (1983). *The experience of old age: Stress, coping and survival*. New York: Basic Books.

Moleski, W. (1985). Developing a housing quality component for in-home services. *Pride Institute Journal of Long-Term Home Health Care, 4*(2), 31–34.

Moos, R. (1980). Social-ecological perspectives on health. In G. Stone (Ed.), *Health psychology*. San Francisco: Jossey-Bass.

Newcomer, R., & Grant, L. (in press). *Residential care facilities: Understanding their role and improving their effectiveness*. Scott Foresman and Company.

Newcomer, R., Lawton, M.P., & Byerts, T. (Eds.). (1986). *Housing and aging society: Issues, alternatives, and policy*. New York: Van Nostrand Reinhold Company.

Newman, S.J. (1985). Housing and long-term care: The suitability of the elderly's housing to the provision of in-home services. *The Gerontologist, 25*(1), 35–40.

Noelker, L. (1982). *The impact of environmental problems on caring for impaired elders in a home setting*. Paper presented at the 35th Annual Scientific Meeting of the Gerontological Society of America, Boston, Massachusetts.

Pynoos, J. et al. (1987). Home modifications: Improvements that extend independence. In V. Regnier & J. Pynoos (Eds.), *Housing the aged: Design directives and policy considerations*. New York: Elsevier.

Regnier, V., & Pynoos, J. (1987). *Housing the aged: Design directives and policy considerations*. New York: Elsevier.

Rosow, I. (1967). *Social integration of the aged*. New York: Free Press.

Sherwood, S., & Morris, D. (1983). The Pennsylvania domiciliary-care experiment: Impact on quality of life. *American Journal of Public Health, 73*(6), 646–653.

Sherwood, S., Mor, V., & Gutkin, C. (1981). *Domiciliary care clients and the facilities in which they reside*. (Vol. 1–3). Boston: Hebrew Rehabilitation Center for the Aged.

Soldo, B., & Longino, C. (1988). Social and physical environments for the vulnerable aged. In Committee on an Aging Society. *America's aging: The social and built environment in an older society*. Washington, DC: National Academy Press.

Sommer, R., & Osmond, H. (1961). Symptoms of institutional care. *Social Problems, 8*, 254–262.

Struyk, R. (1987). Housing adaptations: Needs and practices. In V. Regnier & J. Pynoos (Eds.), *Housing the aged: Design directives and policy considerations*. New York: Elsevier.

Struyk, R. (1988). Current and emerging issues in housing environments for the elderly. In Committee on an Aging Society. *America's Aging: The Social and Built Environment in an Older Society*. Washington, DC: National Academy Press.

Thiberg, S. (1988). Cross-national perspectives on environments for the aged. In Committee on an Aging Society. *America's aging: The social and built environment in an older society.* Washington, DC: National Academy Press.

Tobin, S., & Lieberman, M. (1976). *Last home for the aged.* San Francisco: Jossey-Bass.

U.S. Department of Housing and Urban Development (HUD). (1987). *Housing special populations: A resource guide.* (Publication No. HUD 1129-PDR). Washington, DC: Author.

8

Long-Term Home Care Research

Jill Hoggard Green, RN
Patient Care Management Coordinator
LDS Hospital
Salt Lake City, UT

The population growth of seniors has exploded. In the current decade, the number of individuals between 75 to 84 years is expected to increase by 27 percent, and the number of individuals 85 years and older is expected to increase by 20 percent (Kavesh, 1986). These seniors may be at risk for chronic illness and functional impairment.

Unfortunately, the health care system of the United States is not designed to adequately meet the needs of functionally impaired elderly. Because Medicare and Medicaid reimbursement policies focus on management of acute illness, there is no assurance that the health needs of seniors are met. Couple such problems with the decreased dollars available to reimburse health services, and it is apparent that different approaches to health care delivery must be developed to maintain adequate health care for seniors.

As a result of these trends, interest in the home care industry has grown. In the late 1970s, several community based long-term care projects were funded, and evaluations of these projects have been published (Carcagno & Kemper, 1988; Capitman, 1986; Hughes, 1985). Case management projects and other evaluations of long-term services (Hughes, Conrad, Manheim, & Edelman, 1988) also are significant contributions to the data base of long-term home care research.

In this paper, therefore, I will review selected published studies to summarize what we have learned about long-term home care in order to give direction to future research, including these aspects of significance:

- The effectiveness of home care based long-term care services.
- The outcome measures utilized in home care service research.
- The published research agendas that could direct future research in community based long-term care.

WHAT IS KNOWN ABOUT THE EFFECTIVENESS OF COMMUNITY BASED LONG-TERM CARE SERVICES?

The answer to this question is complicated by several factors. Of significance is the wide diversity of operational definitions of community based long-term care as provided by Hughes (1985), Kavesh (1986), and Shaughnessy (1985). Community based long-term care is often used to refer "to an array of services that include both home and non-home based long-term care" (Kavesh, 1986). Traditional Medicare reimbursed "skilled" home health services, aide services, case management, adult day care, transportation, home delivered meals, and geriatric outpatient centers are a few of the services that have been referred to as community based long-term care (Hughes, 1985; Kavesh, 1986; Shaughnessy, 1985). However, each of these services targets different populations that impedes across-site comparisons.

Hughes (1985) analyzed 13 studies of community based long-term care. To enhance analysis, she grouped the studies into three categories: traditional home care, expanded home care, and case management. Because these categories are not mutually exclusive, they can aid examination of the various purposes, target populations, and outcomes of programs. As a framework for analysis, such categories are particularly useful.

Hughes (1985) defined traditional programs as home care programs that provide "skilled" care to homebound patients. Expanded programs include aide services and/or services received over a longer period of time: personal care (bathing, grooming, dressing) and homemaking support services (house cleaning, laundry, shopping, and errands). The last category of programs (case management) also utilizes a wide variety of services and overlaps with the other categories as defined. Yet case management programs are distinctive because they use a case manager to assess, plan, coordinate, and evaluate a service plan for a client (Weil & Karls, 1985).

At the outset, it is important to note that even with relatively homogenous target populations and purposes of programs, several of the earlier studies were limited by methodological problems. In Hedrick and Inui's (1986) review of 12 home care studies, they stated that:

> definitive answers to controversial questions (may not occur) when 1) insufficient total number of studies exist; 2) the studies that do exist differ substantially from one another in subjects and methods; 3) insufficient information is presented to reconstruct comparable analyses; and 4) methodological quality reveals substantial problems in design and execution. Analysis of home care program effectiveness on (existing studies) permits few, if any conclusions to be totally uncontested.

Throughout its evolution, long-term home care research has gained in sophistication. Recent studies by Carcagno and Kemper (1988), Hughes, Conrad, Manhiem, and Edelman (1988), and Zimmer, Groth-Juncker, and McCusker (1985) employ a more discrete research methodology and outcome measurement than earlier studies. The use of randomization, quasiexperimental or experimental design, and multivariate analysis has increased. Outcome measurement, although imperfect, has improved. Early studies used mortality rates and physical functioning to reflect health status. Recent evaluations (Carcagno & Kemper, 1988; Hughes et al., 1988) have added measures of perceived health status, social contacts, unmet needs, and some life satisfaction measures to make analyses more pertinent.

Because of the changes in outcome measurement, the five measures that Hedrick and Inui (1986) utilized to compare home care programs—mortality, physical functioning, nursing home placement, hospitalization, and cost—will be used to compare evaluations. Although not all studies have utilized these measures, existing data will be compared across each evaluation. With the more recent studies, I will indicate additional outcome measure results.

OUTCOMES OF TRADITIONAL HOME CARE PROGRAMS

Traditional home care studies include Zimmer, Groth-Juncker and McCusker (1985), Mitchell (1978), Gerson and Collins (1976), and Bryant, Candland, and Loewenstein (1974). The general purpose of this program model was to reduce hospital use without compromising the health status of patients (Hughes, 1985). Gerson and Collins, evaluated the effects of an early hospital discharge program with subsequent home care use while Bryant et al., Mitchell, and Zimmer et al., evaluated the effectiveness of home care programs. With the exception of the Zimmer et al. study, which targeted subjects who were chronically or terminally ill, all other subjects had been recently hospitalized and probably met the Medicare skilled care criteria.

In most outcome measurements, there were mixed results. Mitchell (1978) reported a nonsignificant relationship between mortality rate and home care use. Conversely, Bryant et al. (1974) reported a positive impact on mortality rate. Both studies utilized a quasiexperimental design. In Zimmer's et al. (1985) evaluation, 72 percent of the terminally ill patients died within three months of admission to the program. The impact of the traditional models of home care on mortality rate were inconclusive and warrant further testing. This result is contrasted with the results from the other models of home care where it is well established that mortality rate is unaffected by home care intervention (Weissert, 1988).

Mitchell (1978) noted a positive impact on physical functioning. Gerson and Collins (1976) noted a statistically significant return to household activities. However, Zimmer et al. (1985) noted a nonsignificant impact on functioning. In this evaluation, the Sickness Impact Profile, a sophisticated measure of health status, was used making the results more persuasive than previous studies.

With this model, impacts on nursing home and hospital use were generally positive. However, while Bryant et al. (1974) documented a decrease in nursing home placements, Hughes (1985) reported no statistical analysis. Zimmer et al. (1985) reported a trend toward decreased nursing home use; however, the reduction was not statistically significant. Stronger trends were noted with decreased hospital use. A decline in hospital length of stay was noted by Gerson and Collins (1976) and Bryant et al. In addition, Gerson and Collins concluded that untoward clinical events did not increase with the patients discharge to the program. This is of particular importance when determining if early discharge programs negatively effect patient outcome.

Although the studies reported a trend toward reduced hospital and nursing home use, the results were weakened by inconsistent statistical testing. As a result, further evaluation is needed to definitively conclude that hospital or nursing home use is decreased with this model.

Cost data was difficult to compare because of differences in cost definition and methodologies. Zimmer et al. (1985) analyzed "costs per day" for all services. Costs were subdivided into out-of-home costs: hospital days, nursing home days, MD visits, etc.; and in-home costs: visits, hourly care provided by RN and aides, and Meals-on-Wheels. This study reported that the experimental group's average cost per day was 8.6 percent less than the control group. Further analysis demonstrated that home care for dying patients substantially lowered costs. Bryant et al. (1974) also reported a decreased cost.

In the Zimmer et al. (1985) evaluation, patient morale and caregiver satisfaction were measured with impacts on caregiver satisfaction and, to a lesser degree, patient satisfaction noted.

Conclusion

Evaluations of the traditional home care programs produced more questions than answers. Characteristic of earlier evaluations, several of the studies did not measure all of the outcome measures listed. Nor was there consistency in how variables were operationally defined.

Unlike other models of home care, there may be positive impacts on mortality rate, nursing home use, and hospitalization. Unfortunately, only one study (Bryant et al., 1974) reflected the mix of services that are presently reimbursed by Medicare. Evaluations of Medicare certified full service programs are needed before definitive answers can be asserted.

OUTCOMES OF EXPANDED PROGRAMS

Expanded program studies include: Hughes, Conrad, Manhiem, and Edelman (1988), Selmanoff, Mitchell, Widlock, and Mossholder (1979) (as cited in Hedrick & Inui, 1986); Weissert, Wan, and Livieratos (1979), Papsidero, Katz, Kroger, and Akpom (1979) (as cited in Hedrick & Inui, 1986); Nielsen, Bleckner, Bloom, Downs, and Beggs (1972), and Katz, Ford, Downs, Adams, and Rusby (1972) (as cited in Hedrick & Inui, 1986). As several of the study manuscripts were not directly accessible to the author, the comprehensive home care study reviews of Hughes (1985) and Hedrick and Inui (1986) have been used as sources. The author acknowledges and appreciates the work of these investigators.

Expanded programs evaluated the use of aide services and/or services received over a longer period of time. Expanded program models were designed to maintain individuals with chronic illness or disabilities in the community, decrease caregiver burden, and increase patient and caregiver quality of life. A variety of interventions were tested.

Mortality rate did not appear to be affected by the interventions in the majority of studies (Hughes et al., 1988; Weissert et al., 1980; Nielson et al., 1972; and as cited by Hedrick et al., 1986). Selmanoff (as cited in Hedrick et al., 1986) was the only study that reported a positive impact on mortality rate. It is reasonable to conclude with this building evidence that mortality rate is unaffected by long-term home care services.

There was a nonsignificant impact on physical functioning measured by ability to perform activities of daily living (ADL) or instrumental activities of daily living (IADL) in all evaluations (Hughes et al., 1988; Weissert et al., 1980; and as cited in Hedrick et al., 1986). Aide services alone would probably not increase an individual's functional status. Aide service is not rehabilitative in focus, but does seek to maintain the individuals functional status. Hughes et al. (1988) utilized a more comprehensive definition of functional status. Cognitive status, psychiatric symptoms, life satisfaction, social contacts, and perceived health status were measured in addition to ADL/IADL's. This study found that aide service led to better cognitive functioning and reduced unmet needs although only a small percentage of clients (18 percent) were alive at the four-year evaluation. As demonstrated by this study, the use of a comprehensive health status measure is needed to clearly reflect the outcomes of the services provided.

The impact of interventions on nursing home admissions were mixed. In general, it was demonstrated that long-term home care does not reduce the frequency of nursing home admission. Although a positive impact was noted by Nielson et al. (1972), Selmanoff (as cited in Hedrick et al., 1986) found an increase in nursing home admissions. Results were not significant in the other evaluations. The assertion that long-term care home care will reduce institutionalization does not appear warranted with this service model.

Hospital use was not decreased in any of the studies reviewed. Katz (as cited in Hedrick et al., 1986) actually documented an increase in hospitalization among the treatment group.

Cost data was not reported in three evaluations (Nielson et al., 1972; Katz et al., 1972; Selmanoff, 1979.) Higher costs were noted by Weissert et al. (1980) and Hughes et al. (1988).

Conclusion

An initial premise of many of the long-term care projects was that the cost of care would be reduced. This would occur because expensive institutional-based care would be avoided. Yet the results of these studies did not demonstrate a reduction in nursing home or hospital use. Weissert (1985 & 1988) has hypothesized that the long-term home care projects have not targeted the population at risk for institutionalization. The projects actually provided service to a new and growing population of frail seniors. Although these frail seniors needed home care services, they were not at risk for nursing home placement.

OUTCOMES OF CASE MANAGEMENT PROGRAMS

The last category of programs are case management programs. These programs used a case manager who coordinates a comprehensive array of services, including both a variety of in- and out-of-home services. Present were multiple purposes of case management programs including: to reduce premature nursing home placement; increase the quality of life for individuals and their caregivers; reduce caregiver burden; increase continuity of care; reduce barriers to service; and reduce government health care costs (Carcagno & Kemper, 1988; Capitman, 1986; Weil & Karls, 1985). Two large multisite demonstration projects have been evaluated and will be reviewed here.

An evaluation of the Long-Term Care demonstration projects was performed (Berkeley Planning Associates, 1987; Capitman, 1986). Five comprehensive community case management programs were extensively evaluated: The Long-Term Care project of North San Diego, the New York City Home Care project, the South Carolina Community Long-Term Care project, On Lok Community Care, and Project Open (Capitman, 1986; Berkeley Planning Associates, 1987).

Another group of projects, the Channeling Demonstration projects, also were evaluated. Ten projects were designed, implemented, and evaluated (Carcagno & Kemper, 1988). Five projects employed a basic case management model that coordinated community services. The remaining projects used the financial control model that allowed case managers to authorize reimbursement of services. The intended effects of the Channeling projects were increased use of community services, reduced use of nursing homes and hospitalization, reduced costs of care, maintenance of informal caregiving, and improved quality of life of clients and informal caregivers.

Carcagno and Kemper (1988) and Kemper (1988) clarified an important aspect of the Channeling demonstrations. While the projects tested the addition of comprehensive case management services to existing community services, the demonstrations were not a "test of the projects compared to the total absence of case management and or formal community services" (Carcagno & Kemper 1988). Sixty percent of the control group received some formal in-home care, and many of these individuals would have received case management services from the providers of home health care or other in-home service (Phillips, Kemper, & Applebaum, 1988). The use of comprehensive community case management by the control group ranged from 14 to 18 percent (Phillips et al., 1988). It is important not to confuse the results of this evaluation with an evaluation of the effectiveness of long-term care services in general.

To simplify analysis, I will discuss the results of the two major programs, collectively. Capitman's (1986) synthesis of the Long-Term Care projects evaluation and Kemper's (1988) overview of the Channeling demonstrations are used as references.

There were no significant impact in mortality rates, use of nursing homes, use of hospitals in either the Long-Term Care projects or Channeling with the exception of the South Carolina project (Capitman, 1986; Kemper, 1988). The South Carolina Long-Term Care project exhibited a significant decrease in nursing home placement (Capitman, 1986; Nocks, Learner, Blackman, & Brown, 1986). The South Carolina project targeted individuals who were applying for nursing home placement, so the program captured a target population "at risk" for institutionalization. The Channeling projects did demonstrate a trend toward lower nursing home use, but the difference was small and not statistically significant.

Functional status was assessed by the individual's ability to participate in activities of daily living, instrumental activities of daily living, and mental status. Statistically significant program impacts were noted in four of the Long-Term Care projects (Berkeley Plannning Associates, 1987). The On Lok project reported improvement in participants IADL status. Project Open, San Diego, and New York City projects reported significant treatment effects related to mental status. The Berkeley Planning associate (1987) concluded:

> Overall, the findings indicate that community-oriented long-term care provides services that are no less effective than the services provided by existing institutionally oriented long-term care system. (p. 154.)

The Channeling projects did not demonstrate an impact on client functioning. Kemper (1988) concluded that Channeling did not affect measures of client functioning.

The On Lok and South Carolina projects "broke even" in terms of public costs (Berkeley Planning Associates, 1987). Conversely, the San Diego and New York projects demonstrated increased total cost. The Channeling projects also demonstrated an increase in total cost (Kemper, 1988). Under the basic model, total costs increased about 6 percent. Under the financial model, costs increased by approximately 18 percent. The cost increase can be explained by the increased use of community services and lack of reduction in institutional care.

The Channeling projects utilized a larger array of outcome measures. Clients' perception of unmet service needs, amount of informal caregiving received, client confidence in the receipt of care, client satisfaction with life, client morale and social interactions, self-perceived health status and contentment, and caregiver satisfaction with life were measured. The Channeling projects demonstrated benefits to clients and caregivers that were not measured in other studies. Reduced service needs and increased confidence in receipt of care were benefits that clients noted (Kemper, 1988). Increased satisfaction with life by clients was also statistically significant, but caution should be utilized in interpreting this outcome because this occurred with the group using caregivers as proxy respondents. Such results may be more indicative of a change in satisfaction with life by caregivers than clients (Kemper, 1988).

Increases in caregivers' satisfaction with service arrangements and satisfaction with life were statistically significant (Kemper, 1988). Paradoxically, other measures of quality of life for formal caregivers, including emotional, physical, and financial strain due to caregiving, were not significantly affected. Further research into the effects of long-term care on caregivers is warranted to help establish if the lack of results is due to inadequate measures of caregiver burden or lack of program effect. One important finding of the Channeling projects was that the projects did not alter the amount of informal caregiving. Caregivers continued to provide support and assistance to their family members.

Conclusion

The extensive evaluations of the Long-Term Care projects and the Channeling programs have significantly increased the information available concerning long-term home care. Mortality rates and the use of hospital and nursing home services were generally not influenced by case management. Weissert (1988) is probably correct that these services are targeting a new service population. There is some indication that nursing home placement could be avoided with some individuals, if programs target clients who have made application for nursing home placement (Weissert, 1985).

While community care was found to increase costs in some programs (Kemper, 1988), community care is not always cheaper (Kane, 1988). For some individuals, community care will be a bargain and for others nursing home costs will be less expensive.

Clients and caregivers did demonstrate some improvement in quality of life, but questions in this area still remain. Outcome measurement of quality of life, emotional well being, and caregiver burden are less developed and may not accurately measure the constructs (Kane, 1988; Gallagher, 1985). Kane (1988) identified that measurement of emotional well being and satisfaction may have been taken less seriously in long-term care evaluations. Although Weissert (1988) disagrees, it is questionable whether the outcome measures used in the evaluations accurately measured the constructs of health, quality of life, and a caregiver burden. Therefore, questions concerning the impact of these constructs remain. It is critical that sophisticated quality of life, health status, and caregiver burden instruments be developed or refined, if program impacts concerning these outcomes are to be measured accurately.

WHAT ARE THE IDEAL OUTCOME MEASUREMENTS?

A battery of measures are needed to evaluate long-term home care programs. While health status and quality of life measures are of particular concern to this author, this does not negate the need for measures concerning patient and caregiver satisfaction, caregiver burden, cost, and use of other health services.

In the conference on health status and quality of life measures, Ware (1987) presented a framework for defining health status measures. Ware defines health as a multidimensional construct with five distinct dimensions: physical health, mental health, social functioning, role functioning, and a general perception of well being. Physical health can be measured by the limitations in the individual's ability to perform activities of daily living, and mobility. A subjective perception of psychological well being, control of behavior and emotions, cognitive functioning, and the presence of anxiety and/or depression are ways to measure the construct of mental health. Social functioning can be measured objectively by the number of social contacts of an individual, and subjectively by the individual's perception of the adequacy of the interpersonal relationships. Role functioning is the performance of, or capacity to perform, the individual's usual role activities, including employment, work, or housework. General perceptions of well being are measured as a self-rating of the individual's level of health.

Ware (1987) has contributed greatly to the understanding of the health construct. Refinement of his definition is encouraged. In general, however, he has effectively reflected the multidimensional nature of health.

With a framework to define health at hand, development of an adequate measurement tool is the next step. Ware (1987) and McMillen Moinpour, McCorkle, and Saunders (1988) have written reviews of health measurement tools. Ware reviewed 16 tools and analyzed the domains that the tools measured. Three instruments—Dupuy, 1972; NCHS, 1981; and Bergner, 1977—measured three aspects of his health definition. The other tools measured one or two. In McMillen Moinpour et al.'s, (1988) analysis of functional status measures, the investigators identified several health measures. The Sickness Impact Profile (Bergner, 1977), the Duke-UNC Health Profile (Parkerson, Gehlbach, & Wagner, 1981), and the Rand Health Insurance Experiment Indexes (as cited in McMillen Moinpour, 1988) were described in her appendices. Of the tools reviewed, the Sickness Impact Profile (SIP) appeared to have several strengths and may be appropriate for across site evaluations.

The SIP measures "behaviorally based sickness related dysfunction" (Bergner, Bobbitt, Carter, & Gilson, 1981). The SIP specifically measures physical health, mental health, social functioning, and role functioning. The SIP has 136 items and reflects the subject's perception of his or her ability to perform activities "involved in caring on one's life" (Bergner, 1977). Designed to measure perceived health status between groups or within a group over time, the SIP may be ideal for cross study analysis. Bergner et al. (1981) state that the SIP is intended to "provide a measure of effects or outcomes of health care that can be used for evaluation, program planning and policy formation." The tool has been used with the chronically ill and seniors.

McMillen Moinpour, McCorkle, and Saunders (1988) state that the "SIP is one of the most carefully developed and tested instruments available . . . for functional status monitoring." Psychometric properties include test–retest reliability ($r = 0.92$) and internal consistency established with a Cronbachs alpha test ($r = 0.94$) (Bergner et al., 1981). Convergent validity was established by Liang et al. (1982) ($r = 0.97$).

Because this tool measures dysfunction, it does not adequately measure the individual's perception of general well being. Future development of subscales or an additional tool that measures the individual's perception of his or her physical well being, psychological well being, adequacy of interpersonal contacts, and general perception of health could enhance measurement.

Quality of life measurement is increasing in importance. Katz (1987) stated that "the effectiveness and cost effectiveness of treatments must be measured in terms of the quality of life (produced)." Measuring quality of life is difficult because the construct is relative, individually defined, and describes a state rather than a trait (Frank-Stromborg, 1988). Ferrans and Powers (1985) stated "common problems of quality of life measurement are the absence of consensus regarding the domains to be measured, lack of subjective assessment, and failure to acknowledge individual differences in the importance of the domains into account." In spite of these measurement barriers, the use of sensitive measures of quality of life is critical in the practice of nursing. A significant proportion of nursing interventions are directed at improving quality of life for an individual, family, or community. Appropriate measures of quality of life will facilitate development and refinement of our practice and recognition of nursing's contribution to health by the community and payers.

Frank-Stromborg (1988) and Dean (1988) have written comprehensive overviews on quality of life measurement tools and researchers are directed to their reviews. Here I will review two tools that have been utilized in health service research.

Spitzer et al's. (1981) quality of life tool, a short five question-scored index, has received attention by physicians (Troidl et al., 1987). The instrument assesses activity, daily living, health, support, and outlook. Its strengths include brevity and high internal consistency scores with a Cronbachs alpha ($r = .775$) (Spitzer et al., 1981). Weaknesses of the tool include limitations in measuring psychosocial functioning (Mor, 1987). This tool may be appropriate as a screening tool for clinicians, but probably will not be appropriate for nursing research.

Ferrans and Powers' (1985) Quality of Life Index (QLI) is a tool that could be utilized in nursing research. The QLI was developed to measure quality of life of healthy and ill individuals in these domains: health care, physical health and functioning, marriage, family, friends, stress, standard of living, occupation, education, leisure, future retirement, peace of mind, personal faith, life goals, personal appearance, self-acceptance, general happiness, and general satisfaction. The unique quality of the tool is that it measures satisfaction within various domains of life, and the importance of the domain to the subject. Frank-Stromborg (1988) reported that the psychometric properties of the tools "were quite strong." Test–retest reliability with a healthy population was $r = 0.87$, and $r = 0.81$ with an ill population. Cronbachs alpha was $r = 0.87$. Criterion related validity has been adequately established.

Conclusion

Sensitive health status and quality of life instruments are important. In the Wales, Kane, and Robbins (1983) evaluation of hospice care, they measured a nonsignificant difference between quality of life in dying patients in hospice and non-hospice settings. In this regard, Dean (1988) effectively stated "such findings, if considered valid and replicable, could lead to limitations in funding for programs. It is incumbent on researchers to detect differences in quality of life in dying patients."

Nursing intervention focuses on the promotion of health, prevention of illness, and rehabilitation of individuals to their highest functional status. With these goals, it is imperative that sensitive comprehensive health status measures be developed and utilized to measure and demonstrate nursing's impact on the health status of the individual and the community. Collaboration between researchers, clinicians, and program managers is needed in selecting and refining a small number of outcome measures. These outcome measures could be used across service settings and will enhance clinical decision making concerning appropriate health services for individuals.

WHAT ARE THE PUBLISHED RESEARCH AGENDAS THAT COULD DIRECT FUTURE LONG-TERM RESEARCH?

There are three published research agendas that are pertinent to the issue of long-term home health care. Two are studies and the third is a request for research proposals from the National Center for Health Service Research. The first researched-based agenda, by Pearlman and Hedrick (1987), addresses geriatric care. The investigators utilized a two-stage survey research process to identify research topics and questions concerning geriatric care in the Veteran Administration (VA) system.

A panel of 112 VA and non-VA clinicians, managers, patient advocates, and researchers were asked to name and describe three to five problems related to the provision of geriatric health services. Subsequently, a second 38-member panel developed research questions addressing the identified problems. The most frequent problems included clinical management problems, provider barriers, organizational and system problems, patient and family barriers, and ethical issues.

The Pearlman and Hedrick (1987) research questions that are most pertinent to long-term care home care include:

> What are the dimensions of functional, nutritional, and mental status with the frail elderly and how can they best be measured to assist the care planner in assessing patient needs for home care?

> How do the benefits and costs of case management vary with changes in three domains of case management: case manager training and skills, case mix, and point of intervention in the patients health care system?

> What is the minimum data set for the VA medical and health services that is required to provide coordinated and continuous care to the eligible population?

> What effects can be expected from the community-based, non-institutional, long-term care services provided by the VA and at what costs? What are the appropriate domains of expected outcomes and what are the best measures of these domains? How do the costs and effects differ among patient subgroups?

> What models of respite care exist that do not disrupt family ties and are appropriate for families of older, confused, and needy individuals?

The agenda on nursing administration research can be applicable to long-term home health care (Henry, O'Donnell, Pendergast, Moody, & Hutchinson,

1988). Henry et al. (1988) utilized a Delphi technique to define nursing administration research and prioritize nursing administration questions. The expert panel included nursing service administrators, administrators in university hospitals, nursing administration faculty, health administration faculty, and experts located in government, universities, and public and private foundations. From this description, it was difficult to determine the amount of representation of experts from community based and/or long-term care settings. The results of the study appear to be focused on the needs of acute-care settings, but there are some questions that are applicable to community based long-term care.

The questions concerning nursing intensity, patient acuity, classification, and home care clinical effectiveness and cost efficiency are applicable to long-term home care research. Development of measures to document, evaluate, and compare the quality of nursing practice and its outcomes across practice settings would be particularly helpful. Both agendas (Pearlman & Hedrick, 1987; Henry et al., 1988) can contribute to the agenda for long-term care community based care.

The National Center for Health Services Research and Health Care Technology Assessment (NCHSR) (1988) published a research agenda for home health care last fall. Some components of the agenda are directly applicable to community based long-term care. The NCHSR requested proposals concerning the following:

1) Development of studies that link the process of care to patient outcomes with functionally impaired seniors;
2) Identification and measurement of long range patient outcomes in terms of behavioral or functional changes that can be attributed to interventions by health care providers;
3) Development and adaptation of methods for assessing quality of home care;
4) Development of a uniform needs assessment instrument that evaluates functional capacity, social and familial resources, and identifies service requirements;
5) Examination of the impact of different delivery systems and agency management structures on patient care;
6) Examination of the process of discharge planning, and its impact on patient outcomes such as readmission to hospital or nursing home;
7) Development and testing of Case Mix and severity of illness as a basis f or the intensity of care required in a home visit;
8) Examination of the impact of alternative reimbursement systems such as prospective payment and capitation on the process of care and patient outcomes;
9) Construction of a valid and reliable system for classifying home visits in terms of presenting problems;
10) Development and adaptation of methods for assessing quality of home

health care. Methods for measuring patient outcomes need to be developed and tested.

Conclusion

Cost containment is one of the driving forces behind the government sponsored research agenda. Projects demonstrating the impact of prospective payment, capitation, and development of classification and Case Mix systems will all lay the foundation for future reimbursement systems. Nursing involvement in the development and research of these issues is crucial. Reimbursement systems of tomorrow must operate within a framework of health. The profession has recognized the limitations of the present illness driven model of health care and now is the time for nursing to assert a new model. The assertion of a new model can be effectively done through sophisticated health service research.

One area of research presently underdeveloped is the study of clinical management of homebound seniors. The NCHSR has requested studies that evaluate the impact of specific interventions on patient outcomes. This request is an opportunity to evaluate interventions for homebound seniors. Development of interventions for seniors who require management of falls, incontinence, depression, or have alterations in mental status is needed. Intervention research on the impact of services supporting caregivers and subsequent impact on clients is essential.

Within all of the agendas reviewed, there appears to be a recognition of the need to refine outcome measurement and link services provided to patient outcomes. The profession needs to be active in developing and refining instruments that reflect health status, quality of life, and caregiver burden.

The need and opportunities for long-term home care research are immense, but there are barriers. Barriers to home care research are similar to barriers found in qualitative field study. It is the experience of this manager that clients are less likely to participate in studies when they are at home as opposed to acute-care settings. Gallagher (1985) identified considerations for researchers developing and implementing research with caregivers. She found that caregivers required a significant amount of time to ventilate and share feelings. During the course of study, several family crises occurred that required additional services and case management. In addition, most caregivers who participated did not want to leave the project when the scheduled group was completed. The issues of barriers to access, termination, and how much intervention will be done beyond the prescribed treatment are common. Service providers and researchers must collaborate to reduce these barriers and further research that will improve clinical decision making.

SUMMARY

The population of seniors is growing and health service reimbursement is shrinking. Long-term home health care services were developed with an assumption that the services would decrease costs. This assumption has not been validated. What has been recognized is that long-term home health care targets a new and growing population of frail seniors who need services but are probably not at risk for institutionalization.

The impact of long-term home care services on the health status and quality of life of seniors and caregivers has been limited by outcome measurement problems. There are indications that the services improved life satisfaction and reduced services needs, but further evaluations need to replicate the outcomes. In effect, long-term outcomes have not been sufficiently explored. Further research also needs to assist us in identifying outcomes for certain services with precise target populations.

Public policy questions are ahead. Should a program that can increase costs, has demonstrated some but not dramatic impacts on quality of life and health status, and has the possibility of expansion, be funded? The question is obviously debatable. From a nursing perspective of health promotion and prevention, the answer is "yes." Funding should be continued in conjunction with increased research on the program impacts. In Kane's (1988) analysis of the Channeling experiments, she summarized the situation effectively:

> Knowing these facts, we are now in a position to reformulate public policies to design a system of long-term care that satisfies the preferences of consumers and protects them from catastrophic long-term expenses, while promoting the triple virtues of acceptable, quality, equitable access, and defensible costs. . .Nothing in the Channeling results should prevent us from going ahead and trying to develop both community based and institutionally based long-term services in which this country can take pride.

REFERENCES

Applebaum, R.A., Christianson, J.B., Harrigan, M., & Schore, J. (1988) The effects of channeling on mortality, functioning, and well-being. *Health Services Research*, 23(1), 143–159.

Bergner, J., Bobbitt, R.A., Carter, W.B., & Gilson, B.S. (1981). The sickness impact profile: Development and final revision of a health status measure. *Medical Care*, 19(8), 787–805.

Bergner, J. (1977). *The sickness impact profile.* Personal correspondence.

Bergner, J. (1978). *A brief summary of the SIP purpose, uses and administration.*

Berkeley Planning Associates. (1987). Evaluation of community oriented long-term care demonstration projects. In L.T. Rinke (Ed.), *Outcome measures in home care. vol 1. research* (pp 147–161.). New York: National League for Nursing.

Bryant, N.H., Candland, L., & Loewenstein, R. (1974). Comparison of care and cost outcomes for stroke patients with and without home care. *Stroke, 5,* 54–59.

Capitman, J. (1986). Community based long-term care models, target groups, and impacts on service use. *Gerontologist, 26*(4), 389–397.

Carcagno, G.J., & Kemper, P. (1988). An overview of the channeling demonstration and its evaluation. *Health Services Research, 23*(1), 1–22.

Chambers, L.W. (1982). Health program review in Canada: Measurements of health status. *Canadian Journal of Public Health, 73*(1), 26–34.

Corson, W., Grannemann, T., & Holden, N. (1988). Formal community services under channeling. *Health Services Research, 23*(1), 83–97.

Dean, H. (1988). Multiple instruments for measuring quality of life. In M. Frank-Stromborg (Ed.), *Instruments for clinical nursing research* (pp. 97–105). Norwalk, CT: Appleton & Lange.

Ferrans, C., & Powers, M. (1985). Quality of life index: Development and psychometric properties. *Advances in Nursing Science, 8*(1), 15–24.

Frank-Stromborg, M. (1988). Single instruments for measuring quality of life. In M. Frank-Stromborg (Ed.), *Instruments for clinical nursing research* (pp. 779–795). Norwalk, CT: Appleton & Lange.

Gallagher, D.E. (1985). Intervention strategies to assist caregivers of frail elders: Current research status and future research directions. In C. Eisdorfer (Ed.), *Annual review of gerontology and geriatrics* (pp. 249–282). New York: Springer.

Gerson, C.W., & Collins, J.F. (1976). A randomized controlled trial of home care: Clinical outcomes for five surgical procedures. *Canadian Journal of Surgery, 19*(6), 519–523.

Hedrick, S.C., & Inui, T.S. (1986). The effectiveness and cost of home care: An information synthesis. *Health Services Research, 20*(6), 851–880.

Henry, B., Moody, L., Pendergast, J.F., O'Donnell, J., Hutchinson, S.A., & Scully, G. (1987). Delineation of nursing administration research priorities. *Nursing Research, 36*(5), 309–314.

Henry, B., O'Donnell, J.F., Pendergast, J.F., Moody, L.E., & Hutchinson, S.A. (1988). Nursing administration research in hospitals and schools of nursing. *Journal of Nursing Administration, 18*(2), 28–31.

Hughes, S. (1985). Apples and oranges: A review of evaluations of community based long-term care. *Health Services Research, 20*(4), 461–487.

Hughes, S.L., Conrad, K.J., Manhiem, L.M., & Edelman, D.L. (1988) Impact of long-term home care on mortality, functional status, and unmet needs. *Health Services Research, 23*(2), 269–294.

Kane, R. (1988). The noblest experiment of them all: Learning from the national channeling evaluation. *Health Services Research*, 23(1), 191–198.

Katz, S., (1987). The science of quality of life. *Journal of Chronic Diseases*, 40(6), 459–463.

Kavesh, W.N. (1986). Homecare: Process, outcome, cost. In C. Eisdorfer (Ed.), *Annual review of gerontology and geriatrics* (pp. 135–187). New York: Springer.

Kemper, P. (1988). Overview of the findings. *Health Services Research*, 23(1), 161–173.

Liang, M.H., Cullen, K., & Larson, M. (1982). In search of a more perfect mousetrap (health status or quality of life instrument). *Journal of Rheumatology*, 9(5), 775–779.

McMillen Moinpour, C., McCorkle, R., & Saunders, J. (1988). Measuring functional status. In M. Frank-Stromborg (Ed.), *Instruments for clinical nursing research* (pp. 23–45). Norwalk, CT: Appleton & Lange.

Mitchell, J.B. (1978). Patient outcomes in alternative long-term settings. *Medical Care*, 16(6), 439–452.

Mor, V. (1987). Cancer patients' quality of life over the disease course: Lessons from the real world. *Journal of Chronic Disease*, 40(6), 523–528.

National Center for Health Services Research and Health Care Technology Assessment. (1988). *Research agenda on home health care*. Rockville, MD: U.S. Department of Health and Human Services.

Nielsen, M., Bleckner, M., Broom, M., Downs, T., & Beggs, H. (1972). Older persons after hospitalization: A controlled study of home aide service. *American Journal of Public Health*, 62(8), 1094–1101.

Nocks, B.C., Learner, R.M., Blackman, D., & Brown, T. (1986). The effects of community based long-term care project on nursing home utilization. *Gerontologist*, 26(2), 150–157.

Padilla, G.V., & Grant, M.M. (1985). Quality of life as a cancer nursing outcome variable. *Advances in Nursing Science*, 8(1), 15–24.

Parkerson, G.R., Gehlbach, S.H., & Wagner, E.H. (1981). The Duke-UNC health profile: An adult health status instrument for primary care. *Medical Care*, 19(8), 806–823.

Pearlman, R.A., & Hedrick, S.C. (1987). A health services research agenda for geriatric care. *Research on Aging*, 9(1), 101–113.

Phillips, B.R., Kemper, P., & Applebaum, R.A. (1988). Case management under channeling. *Health Services Research*, 23(1), 67–79.

Rossen, S., & Coulton, C. (1985). Research agenda for discharge planning. *Social Work in Health Care*, 10(4), 55–61.

Shaughnessy, P.W. (1985). Long-term care research and public policy. *Health Services Research*, 20(4), 423–433.

Spitzer, W., Dobson, A., Hall, J., Chesterman, E., Levi, J., Shepherd, R., Battista, R., & Catchlove, B.(1981). Measuring the quality of life of cancer patients: A concise QL-index for use by physicians. *Journal of Chronic Disease*, 34(12), 585–597.

Troidl, H., Kusche, J., Vestweber, K.H., Eypasch, E., Koepper, L., & Bouillon, B. (1987). Quality of life: An important endpoint both in surgical practice and research. *Journal of Chronic Disease*, 40(6), 523–528.

Wales, J., Kane, R., & Robbins, S. (1983). UCLA hospice evaluation study. *Medical Care, 21*(7), 734–744.

Ware, J. (1987). The science of quality of life. *Journal of Chronic Disease, 40*(6), 459–463.

Weil, M., & Karls, J.M. (1985). *Case management in human service practice: A systematic approach to mobilizing resources for clients.* San Francisco: Jossey-Bass.

Weissert, W.G., Wan, T., Livieratos, B., & Pellegrino, J. (1980). Cost-effectiveness of homemaker services for the chronically ill. *Inquiry, 17,* 230–243.

Weissert, W. (1985). Seven reasons why it is so difficult to make community based long-term care cost effective. *Health Services Research, 20*(4), 423–433.

Weissert, W.G. (1988). The national channeling demonstrations. What we knew, know now, and still need to know. *Health Services Research, 23*(1), 175–186.

White, D.L., & Pearlman, R.A. (1986). Delivering health care to the elderly. *Research on Aging, 8*(3), 441–454.

Zimmer, J.G., Groth-Juncker, A., & McCusker, J. (1985). A randomized controlled study of a home health care team. *American Journal of Public Health, 75*(2), 134–141.

9

A Response to:
Home Health Care:
Caregivers and Quality

Judith Storfjell, Phd, RN
Assistant Professor
Public Health Nursing
University of Illinois
Chicago, IL

Jill Hoggard Green has given a stimulating and informative review of current outcome studies in long-term home care. She addressed three questions: How effective is home care compared to other long-term care services? What are the outcome measures of home care? What are the home care research agendas which could direct future research?

From Green's review, it is clear that home care research is still in its infancy, although it is moving toward greater sophistication. She concluded that while home care might be comparable in effectiveness to other health care options, this conclusion has not yet been supported by research. However, she mentioned several existing research agendas that could direct future research.

This raises important questions about the effectiveness of home care. Is home care simply replacing care that would normally be provided by the patient's family? Does it have no more benefits than other options? Does it target the population it could best serve? Does home care provide any unique services?

Can home care, in fact, meet long-term care needs? Couple these questions with a government reluctant to expand, or even continue, home care funding and the financial future of home care looks grim indeed. Before a satisfactory long-term care policy can be developed, the effectiveness of long-term home care needs to be measured. The real question facing us here is how to define and measure its effectiveness.

THE STATE OF AFFAIRS

Just how bad is the situation? According to some of the studies reviewed, home care does not significantly decrease mortality, nor is it always cheaper than other options. Then why are claims of its benefits still made? Perhaps there are other benefits besides mortality and cost, benefits such as lower rehospitalization rates, reduced nursing home admissions, improvement of health status, or a higher quality of life for the patient and the family. Unfortunately, few studies have addressed these issues.

In addition to ignoring many potential benefits, the studies cited by Green had conflicting results. In some studies, the costs of care, rehospitalization, and mortality rates were lower, in others higher. In those few studies that attempted to assess the impact of home care on quality of life, no consistent conclusions were reached. Overall, the picture appears rather confusing. It is essential to bring some order to this chaos and begin to study a broad range of potential home care benefits.

Outcomes are the critical measure of any system. After all, the system is set up in order to achieve certain outcomes. What are the outcomes of home care? According to Green's review, there are three levels of outcomes. First, clients have individual goals and expectations for home care, it is for them that home care exists. Second, agencies have outcomes they wish to achieve. Third, standards should indicate the quality and effectiveness of home care outcomes on a macroscopic level. National standards could foster competence on the part of the agency and satisfaction by the consumer. Unfortunately, no well-defined national outcome standards currently exist.

Public policy and payer decisions will be based on the macroscopic level issues on which Green focused. Thus, her report has the potential for far-reaching ramifications. Sadly, if Green's review is to be believed, it seems that home care has no real redeeming features over other health care delivery systems. Indeed, there is some evidence that suggests home care is slightly more expensive.

There are three possible explanations: either home care is not more effective than other long-term care options, or research measurement tools and processes have been inadequate, or the unique and beneficial outcomes of home care are something different than those identified by researchers to date. It seems possible that we do not yet know how to measure the effectiveness of home health care. Indeed, effectiveness has not yet really been defined. Major policy decisions are being made based on research that, according to Hendrick and Inui (1986), has serious deficits:

> Definitive answers to controversial questions (may not occur) when 1) insufficient total number of studies exist; 2) the studies that do exist differ substantially from one another in subjects and methods; 3) insufficient information is presented to reconstruct comparable analysis; 4) methodological quality reveals substantial problems in design and execution. Analysis of home care program effectiveness on (existing studies) permits few, if any conclusions to be totally uncontested!

This points out the need to refrain from jumping to premature conclusions about home care. It also gives a strong, clear mandate to researchers for more accurate and scientifically thorough research.

STEPS TO SOLVING THE PROBLEM

Granted, the current state of affairs is not ideal, but all is not lost. Since home care's beginnings, there has been a positive response from consumers, especially from frail elderly individuals with decreased functionality but who are not impaired enough for other long-term care options. This group may reduce the generalizability of much research, since neither nursing home nor hospital long-term care usually include these individuals. This conclusion is supported by the fact that the studies of traditional home care reflected lower costs, decreased mortality rates, and reduced rehospitalization, while the expanded home care and case management studies, the types of home care probably most utilized by this group, seem to indicate either higher or similar costs with no effect on mortality rates or hospital re-admission.

I doubt anyone would disagree that steps need to be taken to clarify, define, and rectify the current lack of accurate information about the effectiveness of home care. I would like to propose a four-step plan aimed at decreasing the present information gap.

Step 1. Define Terms

The first step in ameliorating these difficulties is to clearly define critical terms such as *effectiveness, quality,* and *home care.* The lack of precise definitions prevents productive discourse regarding long-term home care. Is effectiveness the same as quality? Is effectiveness demonstrated by lower mortality rates? Is quality care defined by the consumer or by the government? What is quality? If quality is defined by Webster to be "the degree of excellence of a thing," would that be excellence in outcomes? It is clear that definitions are vital to any progress. If we don't know what it is, how can we achieve it?

Clients and families for whom home care services are performed are obviously asking for and expecting quality service. Payers need to have quality and effectiveness defined so that they can know exactly what they are purchasing. The providers of home care need to have a clear definition of effectiveness so that quality can be measured, monitored, and assured. Providers also need information about effectiveness in order to determine what ingredients, processes, and structures can best assure specific outcomes. This definition of effectiveness must necessarily precede and direct any policy-setting decisions.

Phil Crosby (1989) states that "Quality is the achievement of specified standards." This is certainly a definition worthy of consideration and application. In this light, I will make a bold suggestion: *If quality is the achievement of specified standards, then effectiveness in home care could be the degree to which specified outcome standards are achieved.* This dictates the need for home care outcome standards, which will be addressed later.

Effectiveness and *quality* are not the only terms that require definition. *Home care* itself has not yet been well defined. Green noted three different categories of home care in her review: traditional home care, expanded home care, and case management. While useful as presented, these categories do require further definition. Long-term, short-term, and acute care also require definitions.

The beneficiaries of home care services also need to be identified. I would like to propose that there are three groups who benefit from home care. First, the patient can benefit through enhanced functional ability, increased quality of life, and increased health status. Second, the caregiver's or family's quality of life could be improved by home care. Third, payers look to home care for its cost-effectiveness and reduction of hospital re-admissions.

Step 2. Measure Effectiveness

After effectiveness is defined, it needs to be measured so that home care can be evaluated, otherwise the present state will continue in which no valid conclusions about home care can be identified.

Home care needs to have some measurable index to indicate success or failure. From the studies reviewed, home care cost seems to be roughly equivalent to hospitalization or nursing home care and mortality rates are very similar. It is becoming apparent, however, that home care reduces hospital re-admission, thus reducing the total cost of a given case. Reduction in hospital or nursing home admissions may be one good index of the effectiveness of home care interventions.

As Green suggested, there may be other desirable and describable outcome measures to pursue. For instance, Ware (1987) mentioned five domains that should be measured to determine changes in total health status, including: physical, mental, social, role functioning, and general well being.

Once we have identified what needs to be measured, specific, reliable, and valid tools have to be developed to adequately measure achievement of these outcomes. Green clearly identified the current lack of tools needed for home care research. Usable health status measurements are just starting to be developed but have yet to be implemented in much research.

Finally, critical predictors of expected outcomes should be scientifically developed so that processes can be moulded to ensure best results.

Step 3. Set Standards

As a natural and imperative outgrowth of definition and measurement, outcome standards need to be set and compared with actual outcomes. This needs to be done on all three levels: patient, agency, and national. Green has pointed out the lack of national, generalizable standards based on methodologically sound research. Since agency standards should, in part, be determined by national standards, the lack of such a measuring rod prevents proper measurement of agency effectiveness. Once such standards are established and accepted and mechanisms to monitor them are implemented, then the effectiveness of home care can be more adequately measured. This requires a uniform standardized data set for home care.

Step 4. Research

The fourth, and obvious, next step that needs to be taken to correct this lack of adequate data is more research. As is evident in both Green's and my arguments, a large part of this problem is the lack of pertinent, valid information about home care and its effectiveness. This could be corrected through extensive, methodologically correct research directed by a clearer and broader definition of effectiveness using reliable and valid measurement tools. A uniform data base needs to be established, based on these definitions, that is standardized on a national, cross-organizational level. Only then can the status of home care be studied and valid evaluations of it made.

Existing home care research has been centered on cost and mortality comparisons between home care and the other existing options: nursing home care and hospitalization. As stated earlier, other indicators also need to be examined. The patient's total well being needs to be tested to identify the major effects of home care. It is clear that when studying geriatric care mortality may not always be a good indicator of effectiveness since a large number of cases may be terminal. It should also be noted that most of the studies reviewed by Green did not differentiate between long-term and short-term home care, which are quite different in complexion.

RESEARCH AGENDAS

The previous discussion leads directly into Green's final section: setting a home care research agenda. Her creativity was evident in finding and applying three research agendas somewhat related to long-term home care. The first agenda cited was one by Pearlman and Hedrick (1987) on geriatric care. Some of the items are applicable to home care but its main focus was on geriatric care in general. The second survey, done by Henry, O'Donnel, Pendergast, Moody, and Hutchinson, 1988, focused on nursing administration in the acute-care setting. This is obviously not directly applicable to long-term home care although it is of some interest. The National Center for Health Service Research and Health Care Technology Assessment survey (1988) dealt directly with home care, yet Green felt that only some of the items were directly applicable to community based long-term care. I would like to introduce two additional agendas for home care research and compare them with the three cited by Green.

In 1987, Albrecht and Perry sent a questionnaire to 187 home care providers and educators regarding home care research priorities which resulted in the following list:

1. Patient classification systems.
2. Resource utilization measurement.
3. Client needs assessment criteria (formula).
4. Cost-effectiveness and productivity.
5. Patient outcomes and effectiveness of nursing intervention.
6. Quality assurance measures.
7. Data needs.

8. Financing of home care.

9. Staffing.

10. Organization and management.

11. Structure of service delivery.

12. Documentation of services.

In 1988, the Community Health Accreditation Program (CHAP) of the National League for Nursing surveyed participants (n = 47) in its Institute for Home Care Research on their views regarding home care research priorities. Fourteen categories were prioritized by the participants as follows:

1. Patient outcomes.

2. Resource utilization measurement.

3. Patient classification systems.

4. Effectiveness of nursing interventions.

5. Quality assurance measures.

6. Client needs assessment criteria (formula).

7. Cost-effectiveness.

8. Data needs.

9. Organization and management.

10. Financing of home care.

11. Documentation of services.

12. Productivity.

13. Staffing.

14. Structure of service delivery.

These two surveys had very similar results. I proposed that the findings of both of these and the National Center for Health Service Research (NCHSR) agenda could be grouped into three major categories:

1. Quality of care issues (qualitative studies).

2. Measurement and data issues (quantitative studies).

3. Organizational issues (structure and process).

Actually, all five of the research agendas fit into these three categories as noted in Table 1. See also Table 2 for home care research priorities as depicted in the CHAP, Albrecht and Perry 1987, and NCHSR 1986 surveys.

Table 1
Home Care Research Priority Clusters

1. Management and data issues.
   —Minimal data set.
   —Client identification.
   —Resource utilization.
   —MIS.
2. Quality of care issues.
   —Patient outcomes.
   —Cost-effectiveness.
   —Quality measures.
   —Effectiveness of nursing interventions.
3. Organizational issues.
   —Organizational structures.
   —Management strategies.
   —Financing and reimbursement.
   —Staffing.
   —Service delivery structure and process.
   —Documentation.

CONCLUSION

As a result of her review of home care research, Jill Green has given us a challenge which I propose is possible to meet. Stated succinctly:

If effectiveness in home care can be defined as attainment of standards;

If outcomes are the best measurement of effectiveness;

If it is important to measure and judge effectiveness on a national basis;

Then it is imperative to:

1. Define desirable home care outcomes.

2. Establish research-based outcome standards for home care.

3. Develop standardized tools which are easily used and are based on methodologically sound studies.

4. Establish a uniform data set that can be used for national research studies.

5. Conduct methodologically sound research studies using these tools to determine the effects of home care on a broad range of potential outcomes.

Table 2
Home Care Research Priorities

CHAP Survey 1988 (n = 47)	Albrecht and Perry Survey 1987 (n = 187)	NCHSR 1986
1. Patient outcomes	1. Patient classification systems	A. Process and outcome priorities:
2. Resource utilization measurement	2. Resource utilization measurement	• Cost-effectiveness of early hospital discharge to home care
3. Patient classification systems	3. Client needs assessment criteria (formula)	• Linkage between home care process and outcomes for chronically ill persons
4. Effectiveness of nursing interventions	4. Cost-effectiveness and productivity	• Impact of hospital discharge planning process on patient outcomes
5. Quality assurance measures	5. Patient outcomes and effectiveness of nursing interventions	• Alternative reimbursement strategies for both acute and chronic care
6. Client needs assessment criteria (formula)	6. Quality as●rance measures	B. Methodological priorities:
7. Cost-effectiveness	7. Data needs	• Classification schemes
8. Data needs	8. Financing of home care	• Case-mix measures
9. Organization and management	9. Staffing	• Outcome measures
10. Financing of home care	10. Organization and management	• Uniform needs assessment instrument based on patients' functional capacities
11. Documentation of services	11. Structure of service delivery	
12. Productivity	12. Documentation of services	
13. Staffing		
14. Structure of service delivery		

If we systematically address these issues, the myriad pieces of data being amassed by home care providers throughout the country can be transformed into information—information that can begin to provide answers to the many questions raised regarding long-term home care.

REFERENCES

Henry, B., O'Donnell, J.F., Pendergast, J.F., Moody, L.E., & Hutchinson, S.A. (1988). Nursing administration research in hospitals and schools of nursing. *Journal of Nursing Administration, 18*(2), 28–31.

Hendrick, S.C., & Inui, T.S. (1986). The effectiveness and cost of home care: An information synthesis. *Health Services Research, 20*(6), 851–880.

Hughes, S. (1985). Apples and oranges: A review of evaluations of community-based long-term care. *Health Services Research, 23*(1), 191–198.

National Center for Health Services Research and Health Care Technology Assessment. (1988). Research agenda on home health care. Rockville, MD: U.S. Department of Health and Human Services.

Pearlman, R.A., & Hedrick, S.C. (1987). A health services research agenda for geriatric care. *Research on Aging, 9*(1), 101-113.

Ware, J. (1987). The science of quality of life. *Journal of Chronic Diseases, 40*(6), 459–463.

10

Institutional Care: Caregivers and Quality

Mathy Mezey, EdD, RN, FAAN

Professor of Gerontological Nursing
Associate Director, The Ralston-Penn Center:
Care, Education, and Research for the Older Adult
School of Nursing, University of Pennsylvania
Philadelphia, PA

Quality of care and caregivers in nursing homes: A most appropriate phrase since in almost everyones' mind these two concepts are inextricably linked. Yet this fact seems to elude many in government and the press who are responsible for and write about nursing home care. Exposés of poor nursing homes or proposals to improve nursing home care rarely cite the absence of qualified caregivers as *the* major deficiency to be overcome. Neither of two recent prestigious and widely quoted Institute of Medicine reports (Institute of Medicine, 1986a & b), for example, make explicit recommendations as to the need for around-the-clock RN staffing in nursing homes.

This chapter examines research findings related to the interaction of quality and caregivers in nursing homes. After an overview of what quality of care is, there follows a discussion of registered nurses as caregivers, focusing on attitudes and behaviors, recruitment and retention, skills and competencies, certification and credentialing, and relationship to nonprofessional providers and nurse specialists.

155

QUALITY OF CARE IN NURSING HOMES

The 19,100 nursing homes now in operation in the United States provide continuous services to over 1.6 million residents who have physical and/or mental disabilities that do not allow them to live in the community (Spector, Kapp, Eichan, Tucker, Rosenstein, & Katz, 1988; National Center for Health Statistics, 1987a). One out of every five individuals living past the age of 65, and one out of four individuals aged 85 or older will spend some time in a nursing home (National Center for Health Statistics, 1987b). The median age of nursing home patients is 81 years. Patients are overwhelmingly female (73 percent) and white (93 percent).

What is a Nursing Home and Quality of Care

Quality of care is a multidimensional concept that includes several components (Institute of Medicine, 1986a). One component relates to the definition of what *is* a nursing home? In the United States, nursing homes are defined by patient characteristics as designated by physician certification of medical need for skilled or intermediate care. Federal regulations emphasize "mobilizing medical, re-habilitative and other resources . . . and the availability of technical services (Day & Klein, 1987). This is in marked contrast to England, where the statutory definition of a nursing home is a place where a qualified nurse is in charge. American nursing homes reflect a medical model, while English nursing homes use a nursing model, with regulations focusing on nursing outcomes such as maintaining an environment supportive of patient independence.

One has only to examine clinical indicators to appreciate the influence of the above distinctions on definitions of quality of care. English nursing homes, for example, use no physical restraints, while in the United States the prevalence of restraint use reaches almost 40 percent. Research (Evans & Strumpf, 1989) suggests that these differences are largely due to the fact that, in England, falls are an accepted consequence of maintaining independence, while in the United States falls are a marker of poor care, and thus need to be averted by restraining patients. Similarly, in England virtually all nursing home patients die in the home, while in the United States, because nursing home deaths suggest substandard care and often trigger a state review, nursing home patients are frequently transferred to acute-care hospitals to die.

Structure, Process, Outcome Criteria and Quality

In the United States, federal and voluntary agencies have developed formal quality assurance systems to monitor quality of care in nursing homes. These systems use a combination of structure, process, and outcome criteria as indicators of quality care (Donebedian, 1966; Institute of Medicine 1986a). Current review relies heavily on structure (the setting and resources for delivering care) and process criteria, the routines, procedures and activities of providers in relationship to patient care. Outcomes are measures that reflect the consequences of service delivery on patients. Although federal regulations have no formal guidelines for determining outcomes, outcome criteria are of increasing interest in the health policy arena.

There is a substantial amount of disagreement as to the relative merits of structure, process, and outcome criteria in quality assurance systems, especially as it pertains to evaluation of nursing care (Mezey & Lynaugh, 1989b). Outcome measures, such as mortality, physiologic recovery, and restoration of function, have an appeal over both process and structure in that they reflect the patient's actual condition. It is certainly more powerful to show, for example, that decubiti are absent or have been reduced rather than that procedures exist to achieve reduction. Nevertheless, there are numerous conceptual and methodological problems in the use of outcome criteria in quality of care research (Shaughnessy & Kramer, 1989). First, changes in patient status may be undetectable or not susceptible to interventions, or may be attributable to factors other than the intervention being measured. Activities of daily living (ADL), for example, have been found to be remarkably stable in nursing home patients, irrespective of either type of facility or nursing and medical interventions (Spector et al., 1988). Thus, expectation as to change in ADL in relationship to nursing care is an inappropriate outcome measure of quality.

Case mix, a second potential confounder in evaluating quality of case outcomes, represents the aggregate patient profile of a nursing home, taking into account patients' ADL, nursing/medical condition, cognitive/behavioral status, demographic/social supports, and length of stay. As a general indicator of quality and especially as an indicator of quality nursing care, outcomes will vary depending on whether, for example, the home cares for large numbers of terminally ill patients in comparison to patients with Alzheimer's disease.

Facility characteristics and time of measurement also impinge directly on outcome measures. Facility characteristics such as size, ownership, administrative stability, staffing patterns, and reimbursement all have the potential to affect outcomes. Similarly, frequency and time of measurement influence what data is captured. Some outcomes are stable over time and can be accurately captured using cross-sectional, "snap-shot," data collection methodology, while others are highly variable and fluctuate between data points, thus requiring longitudinal methodology.

Recent research into quality of care in nursing homes attempts to link process to outcomes measure. The Robert Wood Johnson Foundation Teaching Nursing

Home Program evaluation (Shaughnessey et al., 1989; Aiken, Mezey, Lynaugh & Buck, 1985) examines the concurrence between the involvement of geron-tological nurse clinicians in the care of patients, the services patients receive, and patient outcomes. For a subset of patients, methodology allows for chart review of assessments and care plans of patients cared for by nurse clinicians, the subsequent care provided by registered nurses (RNs) and nursing assistants, and changes in patient status, comparing these process and outcome measures to those of patients not under a nurse clinician's care. Outcomes reflect those thought to be amenable to nursing interventions, such as use of indwelling catheters and administration of psychotropic medications.

The Consumer's Perspective on Quality Care

Quality is also of concern to nursing home patients themselves. In order to determine residents' perspective of quality care, the National Citizens' Coalition for Nursing Home Reform (NCNHR) interviewed over 450 nursing homes residents in 15 different cities (National Coalition of Nursing Home Reform, 1985). Respondents said that staff were "the most important factor in achieving good quality care: positive staff attitudes, well-trained and efficient staff" (p. xix). In response to the question "What can be done to improve the quality of staff?" residents cited (in order of descending importance):

Have more staff.

Provide good supervision.

Find and hire qualified staff.

Give training and orientation.

Increase pay.

Develop good attitudes and understanding in staff.

Give on-the-job inservice and continual training.

Encourage tenure and continuity.

Have a probation period.

The findings of the NCNHR confirm the conclusions of others (Fottler, Smith & James, 1981; Trellis-Nayak, 1988) that the number of skilled nurses are an effective indicator of quality care, and that skilled nursing hours are the most effective proxy measure of nursing home quality.

PROFESSIONAL NURSES AND QUALITY CARE

In 1985, 1.2 million full-time employees provided direct and indirect services to nursing home patients. Over half (700,000) of the total full-time employees (FTEs) provided some form of nursing or personal care. Registered nurses made up less than 7 percent of a nursing home's total full-time employees (National Center for Health Statistics, 1988). Nursing aides and orderlies are by far the largest group of employees, accounting for over 40 percent of the total FTEs.

RN Staffing in Nursing Homes

While an estimated 1.5 million registered nurses work as nurses in the United States (Jones, Bonito, Gower, & Williams, 1987) only 7 percent are employed in nursing homes (National Center for Health Statistics, 1988). A patient in an acute-care hospital can expect to share a nurse with three other patients; in a nursing home, the patient will share a nurse with 49 other patients.

The number of RNs in nursing homes varies considerably (Mezey & Scanlon, 1988). Typically, in any one facility, RNs make up less than 20 percent of the total nursing staff. In many homes, they are a much smaller proportion of overall staff. Only 5.6 percent of nursing homes are required to have an RN on all shifts (Jones et al., 1987). Fifty-one percent of homes have no state minimum full-time RN requirement. Forty-three percent have full-time but not 24-hour RN requirements (Health Care Financing Administration, 1988). In 1985, there were 6.3 RNs per 100 nursing home beds (National Center for Health Statistics, 1988). Federal regulations set minimum RN staffing requirements for skilled and intermediate care facilites. Eighty percent of RNs work in a skilled nursing facility (SNF) or combined SNF and intensive care facility (ICF) certified nursing homes. Nationally, medicare and medicaid certified nursing homes have 6.1 RNs per facility, and 17.3 beds per RN. Nursing homes certified as SNF only employ 8.4 RNs per 100 beds (National Center for Health Statistics, 1987a). In contrast, facilities certified as ICF have 3.6 RNs per 100 beds.

The Role of RNs in Nursing Homes

Given the paucity of RN providers in long-term care settings, their role differs significantly from that of RNs in hospitals. In the majority of instances, the RN is the sole professional in a nursing home at any one time. In contrast to hospitals, which report an average of 45 minutes of RN time per patient per day, the median amount of RN time per patient per day across all nursing homes in 1985 was 12 minutes or less. Nearly 40 percent of nursing homes (7,402) report six minutes or less of RN time per patient per day, and 60 percent of these report *no* RN hours during the past week (Jones et al., 1987).

In a nursing home, the first and foremost RN role is that of manager responsible for establishing, maintaining, and monitoring quality of care. According to Jones et al. (1987), less than 10 percent of RNs in nursing homes deliver direct patient care. During a usual work week, RNs in nursing homes report their primary work involvement as follows (Jones et al., 1987):

Activity	Percent Always Involved
Assigning and supervising nursing staff	64
Observing and charting patients	63
Administering routine therapies	53
Determining patient care plans	47
Evaluating and modifying care plans	37
Administering complex therapies	26
Teaching and counseling patients	20

These finding are supported by those of Colling's (1986) in a survey of 2,244 nurses, representing just over 1 percent of all nurses who designate their practice as gerontological. Seventy percent of respondents were employed as administrators and managers whose role consisted of supervising physical care, coordinating care, and providing direct psychosocial care.

Pitfalls in Evaluating the Effectiveness of RN Performance in Nursing Homes

What factors go into evaluating the effectiveness of an RN's managerial role in maintaining quality of care in nursing homes? In nursing homes, RNs need a repertoire of varied skills and competencies to adequately fulfill their managerial responsibilities. Personal and communication skills are key, since a major task is to develop, supervise, and facilitate the work of untrained caregivers. Competency in managing non-professional staff also is a major factor in judging RN effectiveness in long-term care.

Nursing assistants make up over 70 percent of nursing staff in nursing homes, and provide the overwhelming portion of direct patient care. Data continues to confirm the high staff turnover (over 100 percent annually), lack of preparation (Chronic Care Workers, 1988), and the relative absence of credentialing (Weisfeld, 1984) for nursing assistants. Despite impending HCFA regulations for mandatory nurse aide training (Burger, 1988), the licensure and certification of nurse aides remains in the infancy stage. As of 1978, the typical length of nurse aide training programs was 240 hours, or eight weeks. But even with this amount of time spent on training, standards are lacking as to content, sponsoring organization, type of learning experiences, time of training (i.e., preservice or inservice), or competencies to be acquired (Weisfeld, 1984). Despite the fact that nurse aides frequently move between employment in home health and long-term care, their career mobility is restricted by the separate certification process. Moreover, nurse aides have limited opportunities for career enhancement.

To deal with such problems, much of what a good nurse manager does involves establishing an environment and "tone" in which nonprofessional providers can work productively; as such, evidence of effectiveness is hard to capture using a quality assurance system. Nevertheless, research findings provide some guidelines as to how to structure the relationship between RNs and nurse aides in order to maximize quality of care.

Nurse aides have been shown to prefer a decentralized organizational model, with permanent patient assignment, and an evaluation system that stresses reward over punishment (Waxman, Carner, & Berkenstock, 1984; Mezey, Lynaugh, & Cartier, 1989a). A consultative management style, which favors decentralized, unit-based management and increased staff involvement in decision making, has been found effective in both retaining staff, fostering staff satisfaction, and maintaining quality standards (Waxman et al., 1984; Mezey et al., 1989a; Weisfeld, 1984).

Descriptions of the relationship between RNs and nurse aides represent process indicators of quality. What outcome measures accurately reflect RN management effectiveness? Here research findings must be interpreted with caution. Improvement in ADLs are widely used as proxys for effective RN management in nursing homes (Specter et al., 1988). Yet, ADLs remain remarkably stable in nursing home populations over time, especially for long stay patients. Over a six-month period, Spector et al. (1988) found that 85 percent of nursing home residents had no or only one level change in ADL over a six-month period. Change from dependent to independent status occurred in less than 10 percent of residents.

While ADLs of nursing home patients evidence a high degree of consistency across states, RN employment in nursing homes across states has a high degree of variability. In 1987, the average ADL Index nationally for medicare and medicaid certified nursing homes was 3.4, with a range among individual states of from 3.1 to 3.9 (HCFA, 1987). In contrast, in 1988, the total number of medicare/medicaid certified residents per RN was 17.5, with a range of 10 in New Hampshire to 79.7 in Oklahoma. RNs per facility also varied substantially across states, with a national average of 5.1 and a range of between 0.8 and 14.4 (HCFA, 1987; Mezey, Lynaugh, & Cartier, 1988).

Moreover, the relative stability of ADLs does not correlate with the extensive use of other health care resources. Ray, Federspiel, Baugh, and Dodds (1987), for example, in a study of elderly medicaid nursing home residents in three states, found pronounced interstate differences in utilization of medical care, particularly in relation to hospital use, despite comparable case mix. These findings suggest that improvement in patients' ADL is not an appropriate indicator as to the effectiveness of RN function in a nursing home and is not predictive of RN utilization needs in any one facility.

The preceding discussion highlights the difficulties encountered in applying outcome measures to RN performance in nursing homes. Much of an RN's time in a nursing home is spent in assessing information concerning patients' clinical conditions and making clinical and administrative decisions related to resolution of patient problems. These activities are difficult to quantify in terms of outcome criteria, a problem which will be exacerbated given the increased morbidity of patients now entering nursing homes.

Increased Patient Acuity and Quality of Care

Nursing home utilization data have long substantiated the greater disability of nursing home patients in comparison to the elderly persons residing in the community and those utilizing home health services (Weissart, 1985; Kramer, Shaughnessey, & Pettigrew, 1985). More recently, there is mounting evidence that patients are being discharged from hospitals to skilled nursing facilities (SNFs) more frequently, earlier, and sicker than was the case previously (Fitzgerald, Fagan, Tierney, & Dittus, 1987; Lyles 1986; Neu & Harrison, 1988). While hospital stays for medicare beneficiaries decreased from 9.8 days in 1981 to 7.8 days in 1984, the number discharged to SNFs increased 25 percent, from 2.5 percent to 3.1 percent (Neu et al., 1988). Several studies document that 50 percent or more of SNF admissions in 1984 were medicare patients (Lewis, Leake, Leal-Sotelo, & Clark, 1987; Spector et al., 1988). The probability of a hip fracture patient's transfer to a nursing home increased from 17 percent in 1983 to 25 percent in 1985 (Morrisey, Sloan, & Valvona, 1988).

Nursing home stays now appear to substitute in part for hospital days (Sager, Leventhal, & Easterling 1987). In a study of changes reported by 66 percent of nursing homes in Portland, Oregon, over a one-year period, Lyles (1986) found an 80 percent increase in acuity of illness, and 60 percent or more increase in requests for admission too sick for placement. Use of medical equipment such as oxygen, respiratory suction, tube feedings, and intravenous fluid supplies increased over 50 percent. As a result, hospitals are establishing an increasing number of "sub-acute" care units.

These demands, coupled with moratoriums on nursing home beds and case mix reimbursement, have pushed bed occupancy to over 92 percent and resulted in only the sickest and oldest of patients gaining admission. Spector et al. (1988)

report that of 4,000 new admits to nursing homes, 85 percent were dependent in 5 activities of daily living. Moreover, 65 percent of patients have significant behavioral problems, and 25 percent evidence behavior dangerous to themselves or others (Mezey, 1988).

Yet despite the increased acuity, nursing homes continue to function almost in the total absence of professional nursing, and quality of care indicators continue to reflect minimum standards related to personal care. Current quality of care standards also fail to reflect time spent by RNs on assessment, patient planning, and management.

The Isolation of Professional Caregivers in Nursing Homes

The relative isolation of RNs in nursing homes from nurse and physician supports substantially hampers efforts to maintain quality standards. In contrast to hospitals where a large number of nurse specialists are available to assist with complex patient care, in nursing homes specialists are rarely if ever involved in the day to day management of patient problems (Mezey & Lynaugh, 1989b).

However, in applying measures of both process and outcome, gerontological nurse clinicians have proven highly successful in nursing homes (Ebersole, 1985; Kane et al., 1988; Kane et al., 1989). In The Robert Wood Johnson Foundation Teaching Nursing Home Program, nurse clinician/faculty also provided direct care for patients and worked as consultant advisors to staff (Small & Walsh, 1988). Their role focused on early recognition of illness or dysfunction, initiating prompt diagnostic and therapeutic interventions, accurately and comprehensively informing physicians of patients' conditions, teaching other nurses and aides strategies for preventing health care problems, and personally managing care for the more acutely ill patients (Mezey, Lynaugh, & Cartier, 1989a). Thus the nurse clinician supported and supplemented the role of the RN. Yet, even here, unresolved issues related to scope of practice and reimbursement continue to restrict their employment.

Maintaining quality of care is further hampered by the relative absence of physicians in nursing homes. Fewer than 2 percent of nursing homes have a physician available on the premises at all times (National Center for Health Statistics, 1987b). The most common physician coverage, in approximately half of all nursing homes, is physician availability on premise only at scheduled times. It is no wonder then that a third of nursing home patients are transferred to an emergency room and 25 percent are hospitalized annually.

Recruitment of RNs to Nursing Homes

The preceding data unequivocally support the importance of professional nursing in establishing quality of care in each facility of concern. Despite a generalized nursing shortage, there is convincing evidence that some nurses preferentially choose nursing home practice, and that, if the characteristics of these nurses were better understood, attracting additional nurses may indeed be a realistic possibility.

In nursing homes, RNs are older than are RNs working in hospitals (Colling, 1986). Less than 10 percent of hospital employed RNs are 55 years of age and over, in comparison to just over 25 percent of nursing home RNs. Nursing home RNs also are more frequently widowed, divorced or separated, predominantly diploma prepared, and more likely to have graduated from their nursing program 15 or more years ago (Jones, Bonito, Gower, & Williams, 1987; Cotler & Kane, 1988).

However, little attention has been directed at the extent to which age, educational preparation, or time elapsed since graduation limit an RN's ability to make clinical decisions, therefore contributing to stress and job turnover. One aspect of the Robert Wood Johnson Foundation Teaching Nursing Home Program evaluation will examine if support of RNs by nurse clinicians influences RN recruitment and retention (Shaughnessey & Kramer, 1989).

Unfortunately little is known about job satisfaction of RNs working in long-term care. Colling (1986) reports that satisfaction with both work and organization increased with income, education, age, and experience in nursing and gerontological nursing. In long-term care, RNs report greater satisfaction than those in hospitals. Here, greater autonomy of practice is associated with greater satisfaction.

At the same time, recruitment and retention are proxy measures for job satisfaction. A survey by the American Health Care Association (1988) reports an RN vacancy rate of between 20 and 27 percent. State by state analysis reveals that anywhere from 50 to 75 percent of facilities report unfilled professional nursing positions. When the 6,200 additional RNs estimated to be required as a result of the Omnibus Reconciliation Act of 1987 (OBRA) are included, an additional 21,000 to 27,000 more RNs will be needed in long-term care facilities.

The American Health Care Association (1988) also reports that retention of RNs in nursing homes over a one-year period is only slightly lower (73 percent) than that in hospitals (81 percent). Forty-one percent of RNs have worked in the facility five or more years (National Center for Health Statistics, 1988). However, in contrast to approximately 33 percent of RNs working in hospitals, nearly 45 percent of RNs in nursing homes are employed part time (National Center for Health Statistics, 1988; Jones, Bonito, Gower, & Williams, 1987; Cotler & Kane 1988).

Several studies have linked salary to recruitment and retention (Cotler & Kane, 1988; Jones, Bonito, Gower, & Willams, 1987). Salaries of RNs in nursing homes are substantially lower than RNs working in hospitals. The average wage of RNs employed in nursing homes is $10.56 per hour. Fifty-five percent of RNs employed full-time in nursing homes earn less than $400 per week, in comparison to only 25 percent of hospital-employed nurses. Almost 10 percent of RNs in nursing homes make less than $300 per week; only 17 percent make $500 or more per week (Jones et al., 1987). This is so despite the fact that RNs working in nursing homes have many more years of work experience and have been in the facilities longer than comparable RNs employed in hospitals. In addition, one year retention has been shown to be significantly lower (65 percent) for nurses earning under $300 per week in contrast to a retention rate of 83 percent for those earning $500 or more per week.

Incentives other than salaries that facilitate recruitment and retention of RNs are virtually absent in nursing homes. In contrast to hospitals, nursing homes offer fewer benefits such as tuition reimbursement, and rarely provide opportunities for clinical advancement, such as clinical ladders.

In addition, mechanisms for increasing RN salaries in nursing homes have received little discussion in the literature. Cornelius and Mullinex (1988) have computed the dollar figure necessary to increase RN salaries in nursing homes employing four full-time RNs. For most nursing homes, upgrading salaries to equivalent salaries for supervisory RNs in hospitals would cost approximately an additional $1.00 per day per nursing home resident, an increase that could easily be allocated from a nursing home's operating budget.

Industry spokespeople, on the other hand, have sought to encourage a pass through of government financing to nursing homes as a prerequisite to increasing RN salaries. The effect of previous pass throughs on RN salaries, however, is unclear. Harrington, Swan, and Grant (1988) have suggested that congress enact legislation that exempts nursing wages from nursing home medicare and medicaid reimbursement rates on a one-time basis. Some states have implemented measures to encourage a richer staffing mix, including higher ceilings on nursing cost centers, and special allowances or procedures for the pass through of wage increases. Case mix reimbursement systems also have the potential to preferentially reimburse homes with heavier than average case mix.

SUMMARY

Quality of care in nursing homes is very much in the eye of the beholder. How we as a nation define and measure quality in many ways reflects our beliefs about life, death and aging, and the value we ascribe to those who care for those who are infirm. Many people typify quality as an intangible that can be detected from the minute you enter a nursing home. Others know better. They recognize that the problems nursing home patients face are highly complex and require both a caring and sophisticated response.

There is general agreement that a central factor determining quality of care in nursing homes is the level and skill mix of staffing. Yet how to attract, reward, and retain professional nurses remains elusive, as does how to measure their success.

REFERENCES

Aiken, L., Mezey, M., Lynaugh, J., & Buck, C. (1985). Teaching nursing homes: Prospects for improving long-term care. *Journal of the American Geriatrics Association, 33*, 124–137.

American Health Care Association. (1988). AHCA manpower survey preliminary report (Draft Report July, 1988). Washington, DC: The Author.

Burger, S. (1988). *Nurse aide training symposium: Final report:* Washington DC: The Public Institute, American Association of Retired Persons.

Older Women's League. (1988). *Chronic care workers: Crisis among paid caregivers of the elderly.* Washington, DC: The Author.

Colling, J. (1986). *Findings and analysis of ANA practice survey of gerontological nurses.* Paper presented at American Nurses' Association, Anaheim, CA.

Cornelius, E., & Mullinix, C.F. (1988). *Estimate of registered nurse salaries required to retain nurses in nursing homes.* Unpublished data.

Cotler, M., & Kane, R. (1988). Registered nurses and nursing home shortages: Job conditions and attitudes among RNs. *The Journal of Long-Term Care Administration, Winter*, 13–18.

Day P., & Klein R. (1987). The regulation of nursing homes: A comparative perspective. *The Milbank Quarterly, 65* 303–343.

Dimond, M., Johnson, A., & Hull, D. (1988). The teaching nursing home experiences, University of Utah College of Nursing and Hillhaven Convalescent Center. In N. Small & M. Walsh (Eds.), *Teaching nursing homes, the nursing perspective.* (p. 239.) Owings Mill, MD: National Health Publication.

Donebedian, A. (1966). Evaluating the quality of medical care. *Milbank Memorial Fund Quarterly, 44 (Part 2)*, 166–206.

Ebersole, P. (1985). Gerontological nurse practitioners past and present. *Geriatric Nursing 6*, 219–222.

Evans, L., & Strumpf, N. (1989). Tying down the elderly: A review of the literature on physical restraint. *Journal of the American Geriatric Society, 37*, 65–74.

Fitzgerald, J., Fagan, L., Tierney, W., & Dittus, R. (1987). Changing patterns of hip fracture care before after implementation of the prospective payment system. *Journal of the American Medical Association, 258*(2), 218–221.

Fottler M., Smith H., & James, L. (1981). Profits and patient care quality in nursing homes: Are they compatible? *The Gerontologist, 21*, 532–538.

Harrington, C., Swan, J., & Grant, L. (1988). Nursing home bed capcity in the states, 1978–86. *Health Care Financing Review, 9*(4), 81–97.

Health Care Financing Adminstration. (1988). Unpublished data.

Institute of Medicine (1986a). *Improving the quality of care in nursing homes.* Washington, DC: National Academy Press.

Institute of Medicine (1986b). *Toward a national strategy for long-term care of the elderly.* Washington, DC: National Academy Press.

Joel, L., & Johnson, J. (1988). The teaching nursing home experiences, Rutgers-the State University of New Jersey and Bergen Pines County Hospital. In N. Small & M. Walsh, (Eds.), *Teaching nursing homes, the nursing perspective* (p. 211). Owings Mill, MD: National Health Publication.

Jones, D., Bonito, A., Gower, J., & Williams, R. (1987). *Analysis of the environment for recruitment and retention of registered nurses in nursing homes.* USDHHS, PHS, HRSA, Bureau of Health Professions, Division of Nursing, Washington, DC: U.S. Government Printing Office.

Kane, R.L., Garrard, J., Skay, C., Radosevick, D., Buchanon, J., McDermott, S., Arnold, S., & Kepferle, L. (in press). The effect of a GNP on the process and outcome of nursing home care. *American Journal of Public Health.*

Kramer, A., Shaughnessey, P., & Pettigrew, M. (1985). Cost-effectiveness implication based on a comparison of nursing home and home health case mix. *Health Services Research, 20*, (4), 388–403.

Lewis, A., Leake, B., Leal-Sotelo, M., & Clark, V. (1987). The initial effects of the prospective payment system on nursing home patients. *American Journal of Public Health, 77*(7), 819–822.

Lyles, Y. (1986). Impact of Medicare diagnosis related groups (DRGs) on nursing homes in the Portland, Oregon Metropolitan areas. *Journal of the American Geriatric Society, 34*(4), 573–78.

Mezey, M. (1988). Matching patients and resources to meet patients' mental health needs in long-term care. In M. Wykle (Ed.), *Decision making in long-term care,* New York: Springer.

Mezey, M., Lynaugh, J., Aiken, L. & Buck, C.R. (1984). The teaching nursing home: Bringing together the best. *American Health Care Association Journal, 10*(3).

Mezey, M., Lynaugh, J., & Cartier, M. (1989a). Reordering values: The teaching nursing home program. In M. Mezey, J. Lynaugh, & M. Cartier, (Eds.), *Nursing homes and nursing care: Lessons from the teaching nursing homes* (pp. 1–12). New York Springer, pp. 1–12.

Mezey, M., & Lynaugh, J., (1989b). The teaching nursing home program: Outcomes of care. *Nursing Clinics of North America, 24.*

Mezey, M., Lynaugh, J., & Cartier, M. (1988). The teaching nursing home program, 1982–1987. *Nursing Outlook, 36,* 285.

Mezey, M., Lynaugh, J., & Cherry, J. (1984). Joint ventures between school of nursing and nursing homes. *Nursing Outlook, 34*(3).

Mezey, M., & Scanlon, W. (1988). *Registered nurses in nursing homes. Secretary's Commission on Nursing.* Washington, DC: Department of Health and Human Services.

Morrisey, M., Sloan, F., & Valvona, J. (1988). Medicare prospectives payment and posthospital transfers to sub-acute care. *Medical Care. 26*(7), 685–698.

National Center for Health Statistics. (1987a). *Use of nursing homes by the elderly: Preliminary data from the 1985 national nursing home survey.* Advance Data from Vital and Health Statistics, No. 135 (DHHS Pub. No. (PHS) 87-1250). Hyattsville, MD: Public Health Service.

National Center for Health Statistics. (1987b) *Nursing home characteristics, preliminary data from the 1985 National Nursing Home Survey.* Advance Data from Vital and Health Statistics. No. 131. (DHHS Pub. No. (PHS) 87-1250). Hyattsville, MD: Public Health Service.

National Center for Health Statistics. (1988). *Charactertistics of registered nurses in nursing homes, Preliminary data from the 1985 National Nursing Home Survey.* Advance Data from Vital and Health Statistics. No. 152 (DHHS Pub. No. (PHS) 88–1250.). Hyattsville, MD: Public Health Service.

National Coalition of Nursing Home Reform. (1985). *A consumers perspective on quality of care: The residents point of view.* Paper presented at the National Symposium on Quality of Care, Clearwater, FL.

National Institute on Aging. (1987). *Personnel for health needs of the elderly through the year 2020.* (NIH Publication No. 87-2950). Bethedsa, MD: National Institutes of Health.

Neu, C.R., & Harrison, S. (1988). *Posthospital care before and after the medicare perspective payment system.* Santa Monica, CA: The Rand/UCLA Center for Health Care Financing Policy Research.

Ray, W., Federspiel, C., Baugh, D., & Dodds, S. (1987). Interstate variation in elderly medicaid nursing home populations. *Medical Care, 25*(8), 738–752.

Sager, M., Leventhal, E., & Easterling, D. (1987). The impact of medicare PPS on Wisconsin nursing homes. *Journal of the American Medical Association, 257*(13), 1762–1766.

Shaughnessy P., & Kramer A. (1989). *Trade-offs in evaluating the effectiveness of nursing home care.* In M. Mezey, J. Lynaugh J., & M., Cartier (Eds.), *Nursing homes and nursing care: Lessons from the teaching nursing homes* (p. 127). New York: Springer.

Small, N., & Walsh, M. (Eds.). (1988). *Teaching nursing homes, the nursing perspectives.* Owing Mills, MD: National Health Publications.

Spector, W.D., Kapp, M.C., Eichan, A.M., Tucker, R., Rosenstein, R.B. & Katz, S. (1988). *Case-mix outcomes and resource use in nursing homes.* Providence, RI: Center for Gerontology and Health Care Research, Brown University.

Tellis-Nayak, V. (1988). *Nursing home exemplars of quality,* Springfield, IL. Charles C. Thomas Publisher.

Waxman, H., Carner, E., & Berkenstock G. (1984). Job turnover and job satisfaction among nursing home aides. *The Gerontologist, 24,* 503–509.

Weisfeld, N. (1984) *Accreditation, certification, and licensure of nursing home personnel: A description of issues and trends.* Paper prepared for the Institute of Medicine.

Weissart, W. (1985). Some resons why it is so difficult to make community-based care cost-effective. *Health Services Research, 20,* 423–428.

Wykle, M., & Kaufmann, M.A. (1988). The teaching nursing home experiences, Case Western Reserve University, Frances Payne Bolton School of Nursing and Margaret Wagner House of the Benjamin Rose Institute. In N. Small & M. Walsh, (Eds). *Teaching nursing homes, the nursing perspective* (p. 83). Owings Mill, MD: National Health Publication.

11

Response to: "Institutional Care: Caregivers and Quality"

Ethel Mitty, EdD, RN
Director of Nursing
The Parker Jewish Geriatric Institute
New Hyde Park, NY

I am reminded of a comment Mathy Mezey directed to a group of long-term care (LTC) nurses several years ago, to wit: "We need to teach about tubes and wires." To put it succinctly, that phrase as much characterizes the patient in long-term care as does our traditional depiction of the nursing home as a low key, "medical-advice-available" place where old folks go to live out their lives in an environment of tender loving care.

Any discussion of the quality of care in LTC must first look at the mission of the particular facility. Is it the quintessential nursing *home*? a quasihospital? a convalescent home? a short-term stay physical rehabilitation facility? The question I pose turns on whether we have different standards of quality or acceptable outcomes. This, of course, leads to the issue of operative definitions of quality: patient satisfaction? quality (sic) of the outcome of the medical intervention? sense of well being? Is the patient aware of the nursing intervention with respect to the quality of medical care and, finally, quality of life? All of these are separate but related questions.

RUGs—REIMBURSEMENT FOR LONG-TERM CARE

The nursing home is an objective reality. As an industry, it is undergoing change which is attributable, in large part, to the restructured reimbursement system for long-term care. Resource Utilization Groups (RUGs), the long-term care prospective payment system and the quality assurance system with which it is linked, is fully operational in New York State—and seems highly likely to become the model for the rest of the country to follow in the near future (Mitty, 1987, 1988). Various image sets, expectations of care, and intake/discharge requirements have produced two concepts of quality: quality of life and quality of care. The former—quality of life—would logically umbrella quality of care. While certain fundamentals of quality pertain in all nursing homes, the emphasis on particular indices of quality appears to shift with the type of patient population.

If the patient's activities of daily living (ADL) needs are low, and the medical technology needs are minimal, then quality outcomes focus on quality of life measures such as choice, social interaction, recreation activity, decision making, and maintenance of self-care ability (i.e., autonomy). If the patient's ADL needs and technology support needs are high, then quality outcomes appear to focus on quality of care (i.e., standards of practice).

In terms of the public weal and the social contract, monitored by RUGs and the quality assurance system, the expectation is "to get what I pay for." There is no question that nurses control, are responsible for and accountable for, the outcome. If a nursing home facility intends to provide care for ADL and technologically-dependent individuals (e.g., individuals on IVs), then it must have sufficient professional nurses on staff. The attempt to provide skilled nursing in a facility that lacks the human and technological resources endangers the survival of the patient and abrogates the social contract between nursing and society. To admit highly dependent patients (or, to allow a patient to deteriorate) for the purpose of securing a high reimbursement rate is dishonest, dangerous, and—if the quality assurance system works as it purports to do—discoverable during survey.

A perverse aspect of RUGs, however, is that if a patient is maintained at or restored to a higher level of ADL function, the subsequent reimbursement for care will be reduced. This belies and belittles the knowledge and planning the nurse brings to the "maintenance function" of patient care. It also speaks to what appears to be the medically driven nature of the reimbursement system for institutional long-term care. And while it would seem supremely logical and appropriate for the typical nursing home to employ a geriatric nurse practitioner to oversee the planning of care (and quality of outcomes) of the ADL-dependent patient—whose multiple interacting diagnoses and conditions are reasonably stable—the RUGs system does not provide special reimbursement for this nurse specialist even when he or she acts in the capacity of a physician extender.

NURSING DIAGNOSIS AND DOCUMENTATION OF CARE

Nursing diagnosis (ND) is a conundrum. The language of ND is an unknown to the designers of reimbursement and regulatory forms and systems (e.g., quality assurance) nor is it familiar to or utilized by at least two-thirds of the nurses employed in long-term care. Given its limitations as a compendium of alterations and needs, it seems to fail with respect to the holistic intent of long-term caring. One of my favorite examples of the misuse of ND was an expiration note titled "alteration of metabolism." It has been suggested that NDs become organized into an ICD-9 taxonomy type such that a patient classification system can be developed—out of which resource-care reimbursement and standards of nursing care outcomes would be defined, delivered, paid for, and evaluated.

The patient's record/chart documentation for RUGs completely disregards ND and, in fact, requires a circumscribed use of language to describe care delivered (in terms of resource use per frequency of care item needed). One of the questions in the RUGs reimbursement system asks "what is the medical diagnosis which consumed the most nursing time?" It is as if outcomes of care (i.e., quality) turn on the medical directives of care rather than on nursing "judgement" of the need or frequency of care needed. It also is interesting to note that while the cognitive aspects of nursing (care) do not appear to be reimbursed by RUGs, they are a significant focus of the quality assurance survey with respect to planning and outcomes of care.

Another "problematic" reality of long-term care is that the nurse's progress notes for Medicare (and RUGs) must be "negative charting," that is, a statement of all aspects that are "not" normal, or stable, or good. This kind of note is more typical of the traditional nurse's notes than is the nurse note which we believe is desired by the New York State quality assurance system, that is, "positive charting"—a statement of all aspects which are OK, stable, normal (in addition to what is abnormal, etc.). Indeed, those of us in long-term care are becoming confused as to what kind of documentation of the nursing process is proper—it seems to depend on the piper: reimburser, surveyor, or nursing educator/director.

QUALITY ASSURANCE IN NEW YORK STATE

Computerization of RUGs-required data allows a facility to track medical–nursing needs, patient acuity, patient behavior, patient events (e.g., falls), medications (e.g., psych meds), and rehabilitation needs longitudinally. This is an invaluable tool and method to trigger outcome issues in addition to all the payment and "dollars-worth" issues.

The quality assurance system in New York State, destined to become the model for all states, uses RUGs data and on-site review. Indicators of patient care outcomes are obtained "off-site" via the RUGs data and are known as "longitudinal" and "prevalence" data. The off-site triggers include: ADL status and change per patient, unit, and facility; use of indwelling catheters; feeding tubes; suctioning; oxygen; restraints; contractures; behavioral status and change (as for ADL, noted above); decubiti; urinary tract infection (UTI); etc. The "on-site" triggers are collected by surveyor observation (what I call "walk-about") of patient positioning; grooming; dining room processes; restraint release; range of motion (ROM) and ambulation programs; appropriateness of medication administration and treatments (infection control); etc. On-site, the surveyors will interview patients with respect to their problems and complaints; option to choose (e.g., what they will wear, what time they will go to bed, eat, etc.); knowledge of and participation in care planning; etc.—many of these items are quality of life indicators. In addition, the surveyors will interview the caregiver, both nurse and nursing assistant, with respect to their knowledge of care needed; their offering of choices to the patient; what to do in event of fire, etc. Surveyors also will observe staff giving the care (e.g., ROM, toileting, provision of privacy, releasing restraints, assistance with eating, food intake documentation, etc.). Therefore, quality of life and quality of care are covered.

Patient selection for quality review (in New York State) is randomized and based, in part, on a statistical derivation of quality assurance issues which, in turn, is based on statewide prevalence norms (or "thresholds") derived from data collected since 1986—the start of RUGs. Depending on facility bed size, different norms—or acceptable poor quality of care outcomes—will apply. Are these outcomes of care, these measures, indicators of standards of nursing care? At first blush, it does not appear so; it is not immediately recognizable. However, the infrastructure of New York Quality Assurance System (NYQAS), which includes questions and processes relevant to nursing standards, support the logic of the expected/desired outcome as well as the rationale for looking at the various components of care.

The aspects of care selected by NYQAS were based on input from providers, experts in medicine, nursing, dentistry, social work, physical medicine, and nutrition, as well as on input from patients, previous quality assurance surveys, exposès, consumer groups, and politics. There are 12 areas of quality known as the CaRe (Care Review) Protocols, each of which may have several subjects:

1. Elimination (toileting, catheter, UTI)
2. Infection management
3. Medical, dental, lab, X-ray (includes new admissions review).
4. Medication (pain management, psychotropic medications, medical pass observation).
5. Mobility/physical restraint (includes ADL deterioration, e.g., transfer ability).
6. Nutrition (N/G–G/T feed, dehydration, ADL deterioration).
7. Psychosocial (includes ADL deterioration, room relocation, emotional stress).
8. Rehabilitation (includes ADL deterioration, contractures).
9. Resident safety (accidents).
10. Respiratory (tracheotomy care, suctioning, oxygen).
11. Skin integrity (decubitus ulcer, stasis ulcer, grooming).
12. Speech language, hearing, vision.

As previously described, quality of life is a separate protocol. In fact, several parts of the new quality assurance process are carry-overs from the old survey (e.g., environmental observation, temperature of food and portion size, waste management (linen and refuse), etc.). One new assay is the surveyor review of five new admissions to determine if all problems and needs were identified on admission and followed up. The follow-up process would be expected to include dental needs, lab abnormalities, discharge planning, and the interdisciplinary team conference review. Not only are adjustment reaction and change in condition indicators looked for, but the absence of such adverse changes is a requirement of the psychosocial assessment, that is, the social worker role. The patient who is "at-risk" for physical or emotional changes must be identified, and the expectation is that this will be done on admission and followed by the team in its mutual and interrelated planning, interventions, and goal achievement.

Another interesting innovation of NYQAS is the plan to identify "best practices" such that a facility with excellent quality assurance outcomes can be identified, its process of achieving that outcome described, and the promulgation of said process recommended to poor quality assurance facilities. Whether the "best practice" would become a new standard or requirement for all facilities to follow is not clear at this time.

There is no question that the RUGs–NYQAS linkage is appropriate. Whether patient needs, resource use, reimbursement for, and assessment of, quality of care received is as good or appropriate as it could or should be is under continuing discussion and review.

There is another change in the long-term care industry, the effect of which may be moot or monstrous. The Omnibus Reconciliation Act (OBRA) of 1987 mandated a change of the naming of the long-term care facility from "Skilled Nursing Facility" to "Nursing Center." One wonders if dropping the work "skilled" means a change in the kind, quality, and number of licensed nurses required, a change in the type of patient admitted (many nursing homes are becoming like hospital step-down units), or what. Oddly enough, the federal government is also eliminating the facility-type designation of "Intermediate Care Facility" and has developed requirements for numbers of nurses needed per bed capacity. In long-term care, there is more than a semantic difference in the calculation of "nursing care hours" and "skilled nursing hours"—this needs to be made clear to our legislators and regulators.

As a marker of care, falls would appear to be a superior index. In Great Britain, a patient fall is not an indicator of poor care; it is, however, in the United States. In part, the issue is related to the use of physical restraints. Given the notoriety of restraint use as a behavior modifier and staff convenience, there "is" a proper use of restraints. A hip fracture (or the like) is life threatening due to the enforced immobility and possible need for an indwelling catheter. Obviously, correct patient assessment and risk management is necessary, notwithstanding that we are a more litigious society than our English confreres.

NURSING: PROFESSIONAL AND NONPROFESSIONAL STAFF NEEDS

What is the task of professional nursing in long-term care? In describing RUGs–NYQAS, part of the task, albeit imposed on us from without, is clearly defined. Using the three cardinals of our profession—education, practice, and research—efforts to provide quality are evident. But first, we need to have nurses in the setting. The 1985–1987 study of RNs in long-term care with respect to their characteristics, recruitment and retention, indicated that salary and benefits (including tuition reimbursement and access to education) and longevity reimbursement ("award") were key issues. The long-term care nurse is not dissimilar from the hospital nurse, although he or she tends to be predominantly diploma educated, older, and female. An interesting, unexpected, and dismaying finding of this survey ("n" of approximately 2,500 nurses representing approximately 100,000 nurses in long-term care) was that the master's prepared clinician (as supervisor) was less valued than a supervisor who "knew her job." Also, being part of a clinical campus site or having students in the facility was apparently not valued by the respondents.

The gerontological education needs of the nursing student as well as practitioner are well known yet we see minimal efforts at broadening the time spent, scope or depth of the supervised clinical experience. Anecdotal reports describe that while the nursing student's attitude toward and perception of the geriatric patient improves after exposure, there is no surge of applicants for employment in the long-term care setting. The experience of the Robert Wood Johnson Project (of placing geriatric nurse practitioners (GNPs) in nursing homes) was described as "highly successful" but we don't know "at what" and if it can be replicated without significant dollars and doers.

Nursing Assistants

Since two-thirds of the nursing staff in a nursing home are nursing assistants (NAs), their education and training needs have been well recognized by the industry. While additional reimbursement was provided in order to hire educators/"trainers," it was not sufficient to meet their didactic and supervisory needs. Federal regulation now requires that all NAs receive a minimum of 80 hours (in New York State: 100 hours) of training after which a written and "observation" examination must be taken and passed. The NA is then certified and becomes part of a NA registry. The examination is still under development as is the curriculum, and includes communication skills, direct care procedures, knowledge of diseases and disabilities of the elderly, vital signs, and so on.

A long-term care nurse relies on the hands, eyes, ears, and mouth of the NA to provide 70 percent of patient care. It speaks to the enormity of the problem that the literacy proficiency level of the examination has been reduced from a 6th to a 3rd grade level. If the written examination is failed, the NA may take it two more times, written or oral. The distrust with which the government (regulatory agencies) views long-term care is exemplified by the requirement that neither the clinical observation/test nor written examination can be given by the facility's own educator. The overall perception of the nursing home sector as second-class again is exemplified by the educator and the education program language, that is, "train the trainer" and "training program."

QUALITY ASSURANCE PROCESSES

It is unlikely that there is any nursing home that has no quality assurance processes in place. Some may be pure audit (paper) trail, that is, find the error, fix it. Others start as a paper audit, fix it, but include an education intervention step to correct unacceptable or poor practice. Several examples follow:

1. Nasogastric and Gastrostomy Tube: date of original insertion, reason; current weight, gain or loss; ideal body weight; feeding amount, gravity or pump, continuous or intermittent; mitten restraints; (aspiration) pneumonia.

    With respect to enteral feeding, while it might be expected or reasonable to need mitten restraints for a patient with a N/G tube, it would be reasonable to ask why mitts are used for patients with a G/T.

    If the patient is mentally alert, one should consider if continuous feeding during the night be substituted for intermittent feedings which may be preventing the patient from social activities or interactions?

    A dysphagia evaluation should be done prior to tube insertion and at some interval thereafter. A study conducted several years ago at my facility indicated that there is no difference in the incidence of aspiration pneumonia in patients with N/G or G/T. Given that a G/T is more socially acceptable, has it been considered for "X" patient with a N/G tube? (Bear in mind that RUGs give a higher reimbursement for a patient with a N/G tube!).

    Has a dysphagia evaluation been done?

2. Medical Transcription Audit: error identified. Was it simply corrected or was nurse spoken to with reeducation needs: process of orders transcription? Is time management an issue; that is, the nurse was rushing, the physician got in the orders late; is the nurse aware of the potential danger? Is the nurse aware of the fundamental pharmacologic action of the medication? If a medication was held due to vital signs, how many times was it held? At what point was the physician notified?

3. Accidents/Risk Management Review reveals that many patients are falling in a self-toileting attempt. Is this related to staff meal break, change of shift, pre-meal toileting, call bells being answered, a staff conference held right after a meal, or lack of patient teaching for self-transfers? Patients are falling out of wheel chairs yet restraints

are on. Was it properly applied? Did the nursing assistant give a return demonstration of proper application?

As we all know, it is one thing to collect the data, it is quite another to convert it into information that explains something. In addition to the above, at my facility some quality assurance processes we look at include:

1. Indwelling and external catheter use/justification, UTI, relation to obesity and ability to toilet transfer; presence of decubitus, neurogenic bladder, urometrics, etc.
2. Seizure disorders: is patient wheelchair mobile? (mouthbit on chair?)
3. Food intake documentation in relation to weight change.
4. Random sample orders audit.
5. Psychotropic medication utilization.
6. Relationship of the nursing care plan to goal achievement.
7. Decubitus presence, management, and nutritional status.
8. NA signatures verifying care given; bowel movements.
9. Environment: toilet bar safety; bed wheel locks; call bell attachment to bed; personal care items labeled with patient name.

One of the difficult aspects of quality assurance is to convince and reassure the professional and nonprofessional staff that quality assurance is not simply an "I gotcha!" process but a process designed as peer support to help identify problems and learning needs. Depending on the nurse's (mis)conceptions about what "autonomy" really means, and the level of trust which prevails, a quality assurance system can be sabotaged. Of course, the nurse who goofed is told by his or her colleague, but the extent and breadth of the goofs are hidden from the supervisors and educators perhaps out of fear of retaliation or poor performance review.

In the context of quality assurance, then, peer review has been shown to be effective. It also would be an excellent student clinical placement or preceptorship for a student to identify a quality assurance issue (or standard), construct an assessment tool based on standards of practice with measurement criteria, select an outcome standard, test it, and share it. The findings may reveal a practice issue requiring educational remediation, or an operational issue requiring system restructure, or a staffing level/number issue. This (and others like it) becomes a tool for the nursing director in his or her continuous effort to demand the resources needed!

QUALITY ASSURANCE LONG-TERM CARE

With respect to research on quality assurance outcomes in nursing homes, a traditional dearth of literature exists. A study to determine whether newly admitted nursing home patients' experience of stress was related to (external surveyor) judgement of the quality of the nursing home revealed that patients placed in poorer quality nursing homes had a greater need for "tender loving care" across the measured time periods. In contrast, patients in "good" nursing homes expressed more concern about the medical care than they did about the tender loving care provided. These patients expected less stress on admission from "relationship" issues but, as they remained in the facility, their stress level in this area increased (Stein, Linn, & Stein, 1986).

An assay of (1) nurses' perceptions of what constitutes indicators of quality of life (QOL) and (2) nurses' observed frequency of their staff's QOL behaviors, conducted by one of my rehabiliation nurses at a large urban long-term care facility, indicated that while the nurses' overall perception of QOL indices was high, the observed frequency of QOL behaviors was just midline.

A study reported by Huss, Buckwelter, and Stolley (1988) found that nursing's impact on patient "satisfaction with life" in an intermedicate care institutional setting was impacted by the nurse acting as a "health promoter and confidant." It appeared that an individual's perceived health status was closely related to his or her life satisfaction. Because RUGs reimburse more for high dependency patients while overlooking "patient counseling," a pertinent question rises: What kind of impact can the nurse really have on a patient's quality of life and satisfaction?

The final study I commend to your attention asked the question of "who" sets nursing standards: the profession itself, the setting, or the legal environment (Young, 1988). Six dependent variables, selected as indicators of nursing standards, were drawn from the American Nurses' Association minimum expectations of nursing practice (e.g., performing physical and psychosocial examination, performing nursing diagnosis, patient teaching, etc.). The four variables selected as indicators of the profession's influence on standards of practice included: nursing degree earned, current specialist certification, continuing education, and years since the nurse earned the nursing degree. Indicators of influence of the practice setting (place of employment) were also treated as independent variables; they were inpatient or outpatient setting and the type of organization (i.e., for-profit, private not-for-profit, or government).

Young's (1988) findings, in brief, were:

1. The type of service provided (inpatient versus outpatient) was significantly related to the frequency of nursing function.

2. Physical and psychosocial examination frequency was similar to nursing diagnosis performance: NDs were performed more frequently in inpatient settings. The influence of service type diminished with the nurses' increased continuing education, BS degree, and recent formal nursing education.

3. Patient teaching occurred more frequently in the outpatient setting and was done more frequently by nurses with continuing education, a recent degree, and by nurses who were not specialty certified. Formal nursing education programs did not appear to influence patient teaching performance.

4. Nursing diagnosis performance appeared to be related more with baccalaureate degree nurses than master's prepared nurses.

5. Certification was positively related to patient examination but did not appear to influence nursing diagnosis performance. It was negatively and significantly correlated with patient education. Young's (1988) overall conclusion, after analyzing the responses of over 75,000 nurses (in Illinois from a pool of over 110,000 nurses), was that the profession, through its formal education and continuing education programs, had a greater influence on nursing standards than did the type of service, work setting, and specialty certification.

The implications of this study attest to the need for tuition support, educational access, and scheduling for staff development.

While a variety of quality assurance studies may be suggested, we clearly need to look at the different types of nursing professional (and nonprofessional) with respect to outcomes of care in the institutional setting. Differentiated practice models will require a quality assurance component for evaluation. Computerization of patient data and nursing information systems similarly require a quality assurance processing and audit trail.

It is my conviction that quality assurance processes are the *sine qua non* of the nursing profession, as well as its social contract. For many reasons, nursing is not, nor can it be, timorous in identifying poor practice and improving the performance of its practitioners (nurses) and the people who work under their guidance and tutelage.

REFERENCES

Huss, M.J., Buckwalter, K.C., & Stolley, J. (1988). Nursing's impact on life satisfaction. *Journal of Gerontological Nursing, 14*(5), 31–36.

Mitty, E. (1987). PPS in long-term care. *Nursing & Health Care, 8*(1), 14–21.

Mitty, E. (1988). RUGs: DRGs move to long-term care. *Nursing Clinics of North America, 23*(3), 539–557.

Stein S., Linn M.W., & Stein E.M. (1986). Patient's perceptions of nursing home stress related to quality of care. *The Gerontologist, 26*(4), 424–430.

Young, W.B. (1988). Who sets nursing standards: The nursing profession or the employment setting? *Nursing Administration Quarterly, 12*(2), 78–86.